THE
WALKING
EFFECT

Karl Henry is one of Ireland's most recognised personal trainers and is well known from his time on RTÉ's *Operation Transformation*. Karl has a BSc in Sports Science and Sports Management from University College Dublin, as well as three personal training qualifications: ACE, AABS and PN1.

THE MAGIC OF WALKING
FOR WELL-BEING AND THE BEST
PLACES IN IRELAND TO DO IT

THE WALKING EFFECT

KARL HENRY

GILL BOOKS

Gill Books
Hume Avenue
Park West
Dublin 12
www.gillbooks.ie

Gill Books is an imprint of M.H. Gill and Co.

978 18045 8340 1

Designed by Graham Thew © Gill Books
Print origination by Alba Esteban (@alesturadesign)
Edited by Jane Rogers
Proofread by Esther Ní Dhonnacha
Illustrations by Lydia Moran
Printed and bound by Firmengruppe APPL, Germany
This book is typeset in Dante MT Pro 10/15 and Gotham.

This book is not intended as a substitute for the medical advice of a physician. The reader should consult a doctor or mental health professional if they feel it necessary.

Hiking is a risk activity. The author and publishers accept no responsibility for any injury, loss or inconvenience sustained by anyone using this book.

The paper used in this book comes from the wood pulp of sustainably managed forests.

To the best of our knowledge, this book complies in full with the requirements of the General Product Safety Regulation (GPSR). For further information and help with any safety queries, please contact us at productsafety@gill.ie.

A CIP catalogue record for this book is available from the British Library.

5 4 3 2 1

———

I have loved spending the 25 years of my career so far working with my clients, followers, listeners and viewers as they strive to improve their health and wellness. This book is for everyone who has joined me on that journey. Here's to the next 25!

———

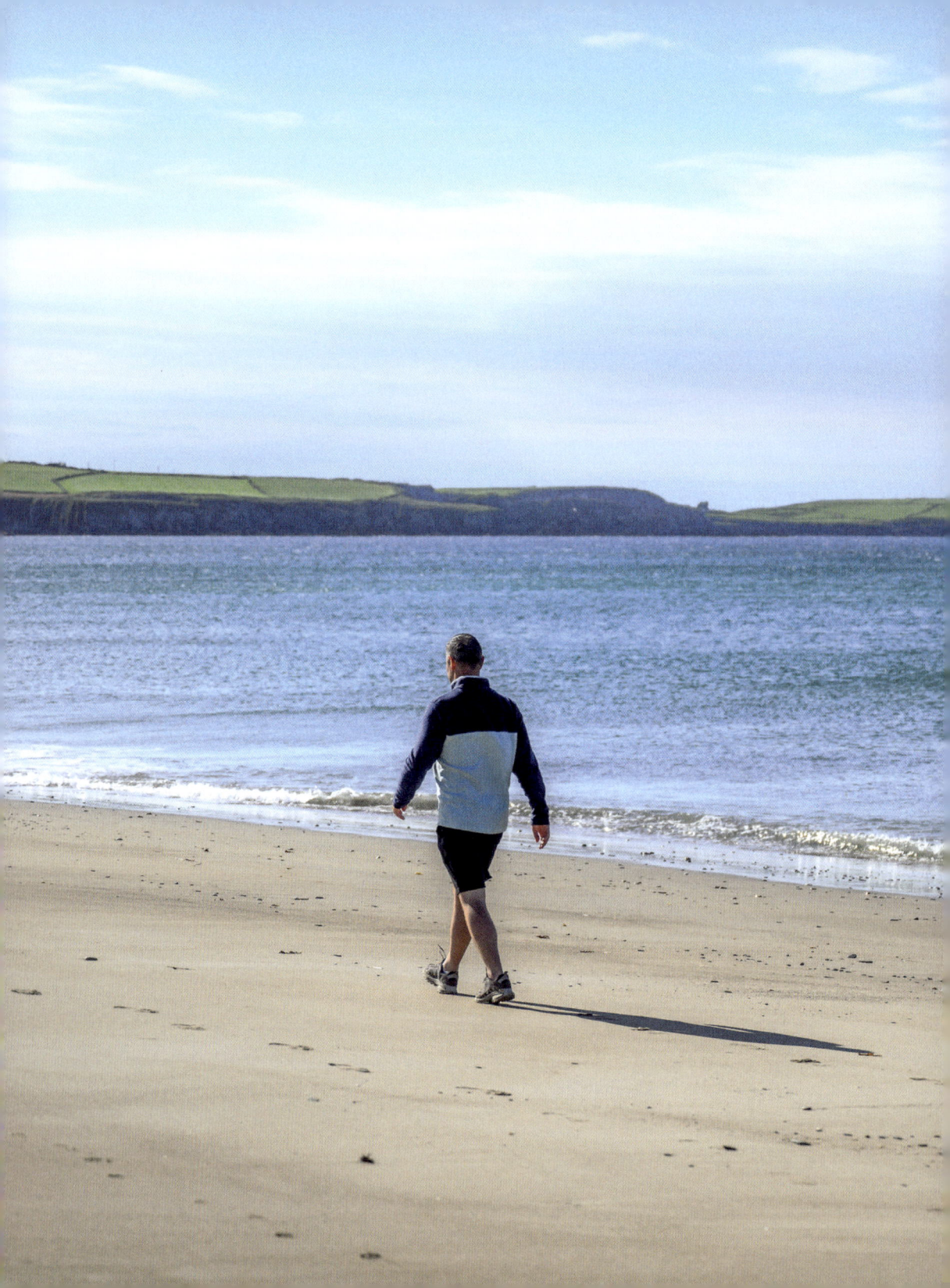

CONTENTS

CHAPTER THREE: WHAT TO WEAR AND WHAT TO BRING

CHAPTER FOUR: NATURE – THE SUPERPOWER YOU DIDN'T KNOW EXISTED

CHAPTER FIVE: SOME OF MY FAVOURITE WALKS IN IRELAND

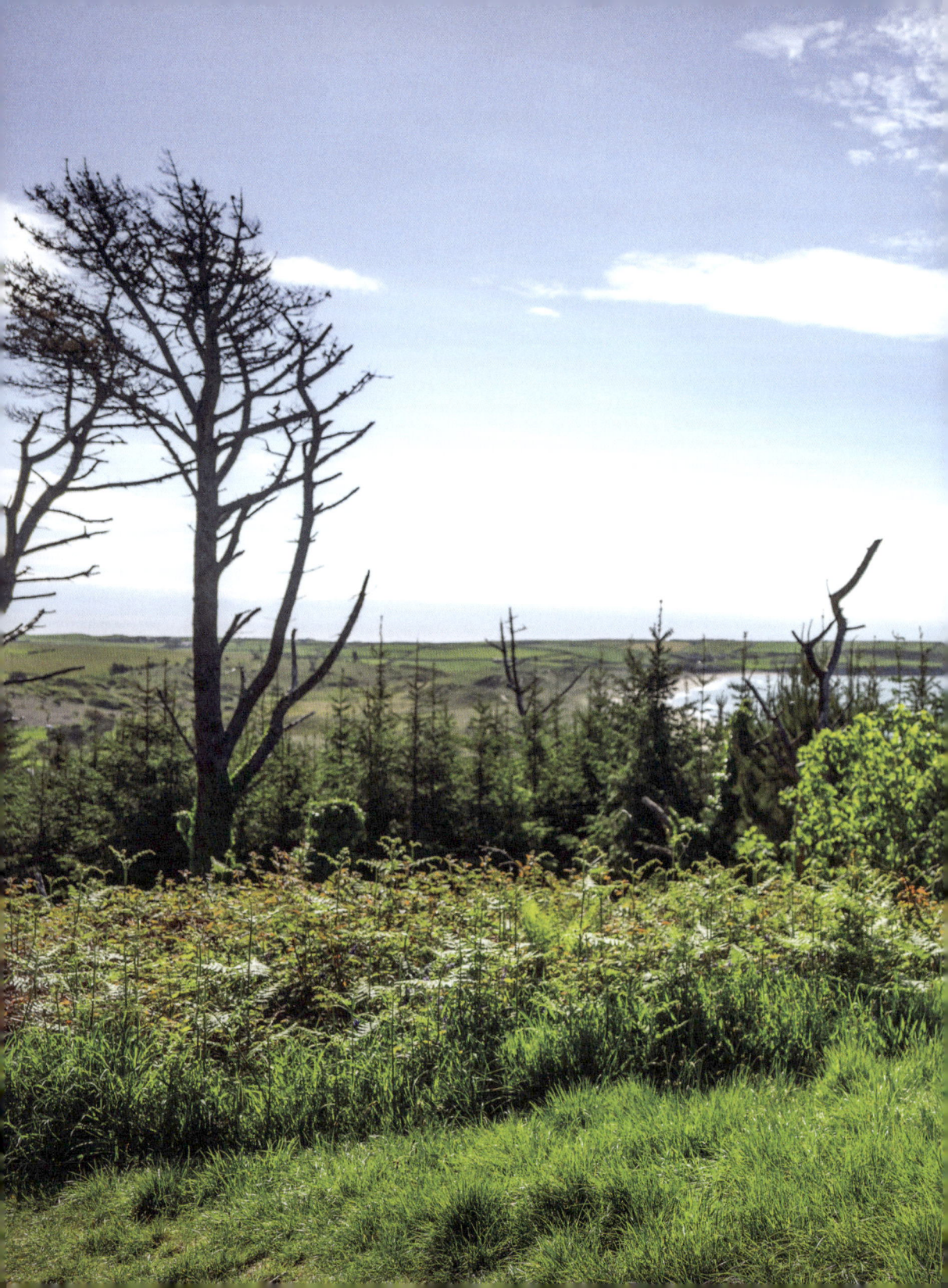

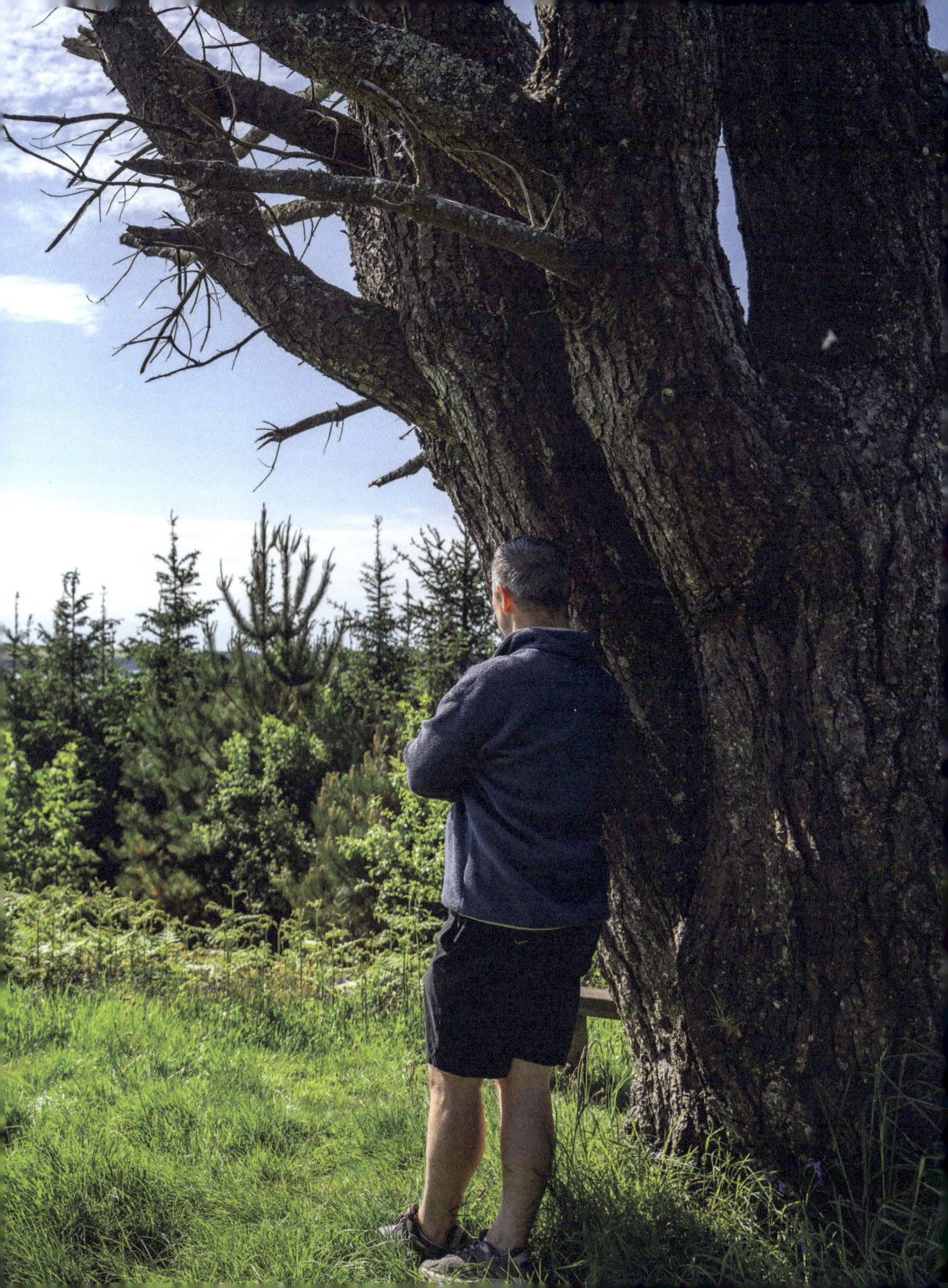

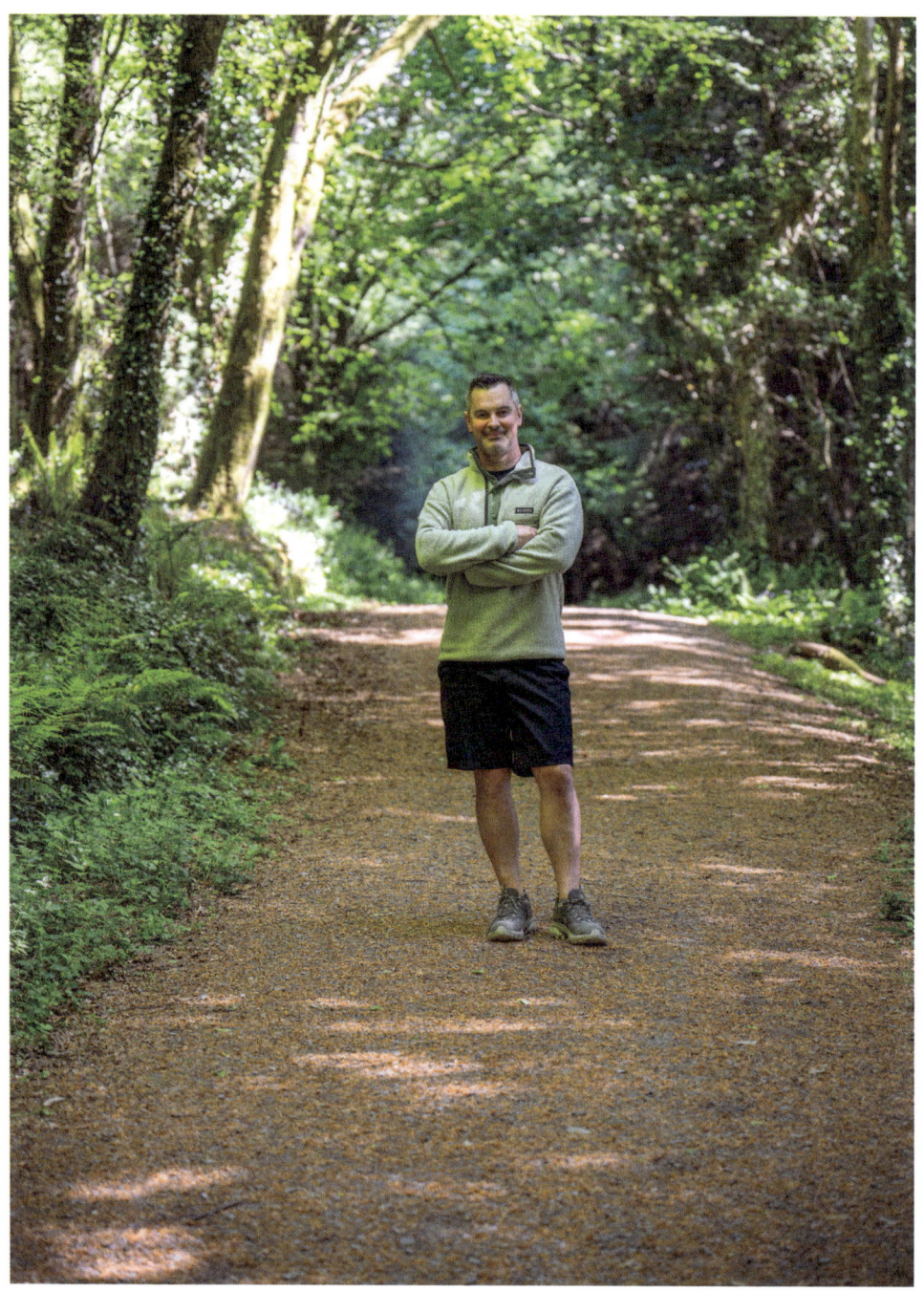

INTRODUCTION

Welcome to *The Walking Effect*. I am so excited that you have picked up this book! Over the last 25 years, in my work helping people to improve their health and wellbeing, walking has been the one constant tool I have used. The impact it has on people's health never ceases to amaze me.

Walking is so simple, so obvious, so accessible and offers so many benefits, but I think it is something we have almost forgotten about. The benefits, the impact and the simplicity. Walking is our very own therapy and medicine. Our way to de-stress, to stay strong, to be mindful ... to just be.

We are always looking for ways to get healthy – the magic pill, the latest diet, the new movement fad – but the further we look the further we tend to fall. Fads fail. Quick fixes are short-lived. Complicated has become the new simple. With this book, I want to change that. Over the course of my career I have seen every quick fix come and go. My mission is to make exercise simple and accessible, and to show people just how easy it is.

I believe it is time for us all to take a deep breath, to go back to basics and to understand the incredible power that is walking. Although it is something we have done forever, it is something we are now doing less and less. In this book I am going to delve into the world of walking. I'm going to show you just why it is so incredible and what it is going to do for you. I'll give you all the information you need to make walking your own personal superpower!

WHY I WALK

I love to walk. It calms me down. It takes me away from my phone. It makes me take in the world around me. It lowers my stress levels, helps me work better and makes me a nicer person to be around. It's when I'm walking that I get some of my best ideas, including the idea for this book.

We are all permanently distracted. When was the last time that you just sat in nature and properly took in your surroundings? We all struggle to be present, now more than ever. But every now and again, when I take the time, I am blown away by the colour of water, by the singing of birds, by the light in the trees. Being honest, walking just always makes me feel better. I walk whenever I can, wherever I can. If there's a chance to walk between meetings, I'll always take it. When I get off the train in Dublin every time I travel up for work, I walk to my meetings or events. When I am working at home and stressed, I just take some time out to stroll around the fields and take in the scenes around me. Recently we took our first group on the Camino de Santiago, and over five days we walked 115km through the Spanish countryside. The impact on the people in the group of just being present, walking and taking it all in blew me away. It was transformational.

WHY I BELIEVE WALKING IS SUCH GOOD EXERCISE

People often ask me why I talk more about walking than running. I love running, but I know that not everyone does. Most people prefer to walk and – as running and walking do pretty much the same thing – I would always advise you to do what you like better. Walking is easier on the joints, less likely to cause injury and suitable for almost everyone, whatever your age and stage of life.

But it's worth remembering that if you're going to walk as your main exercise, intensity is key. You need to be working hard enough to get out of breath but should still be able to hold a conversation. It's about getting your heart rate up. As you get fitter, as with all forms of exercise, you need to keep challenging yourself. Track what you're doing and once you hit your goal, set yourself a new target. That could be climbing the tallest peak in your county, walking a 5k or even achieving 10,000 steps. The goal itself doesn't matter; what is most important is setting that goal and then, when you achieve it, rewarding yourself with something. The goal–reward habit is a great one to keep you motivated all year round.

Also remember that you need to change your route as often as you can. Use flatter routes to get your pace up, and use hilly routes to improve your fitness. Think about why you're walking and tailor the routes to suit you. And use walking as an excuse to explore.

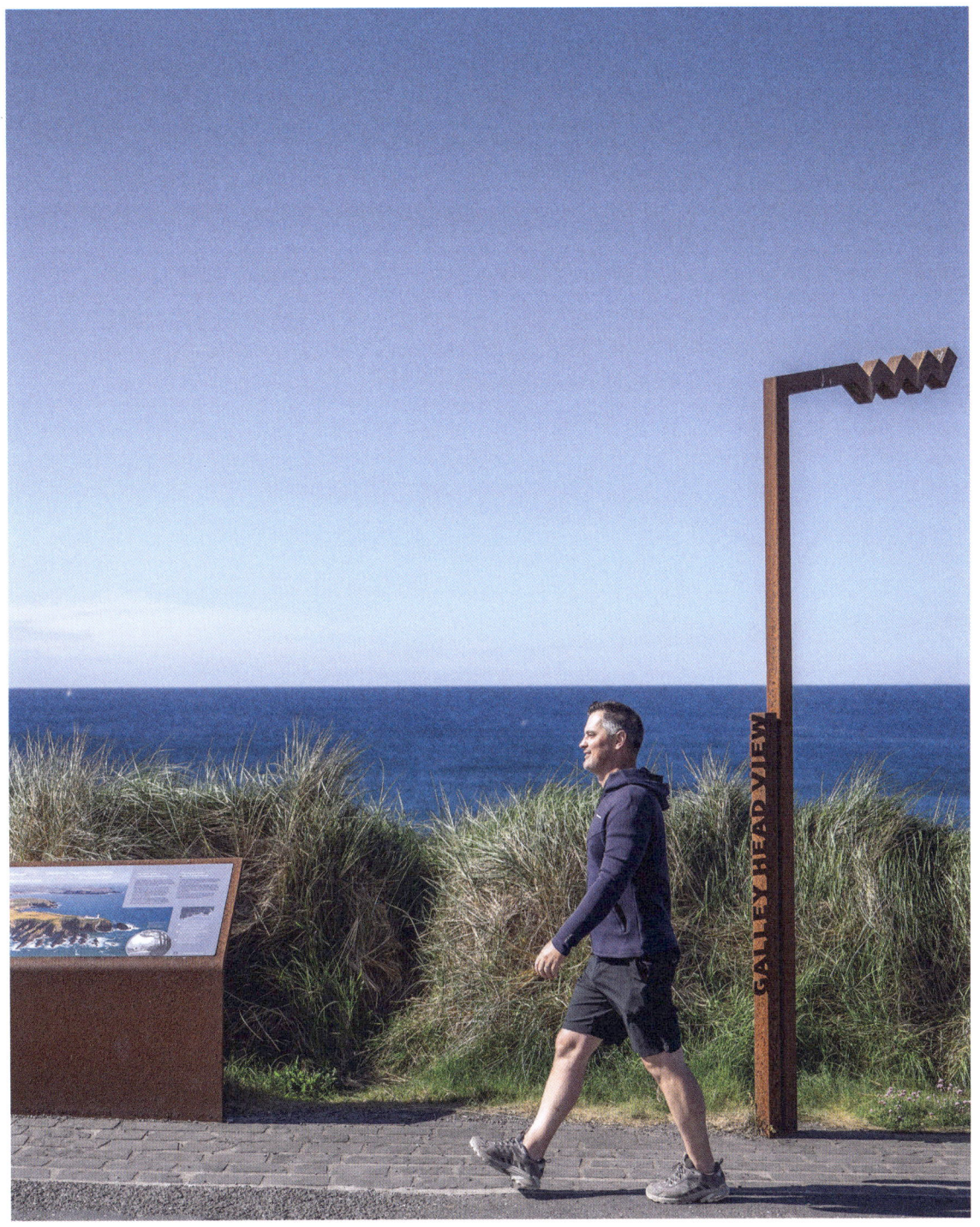

HOW TO USE THIS BOOK

So many self-help books offer complicated ways to improve your mental and physical health, promising incredible transformations within a really short space of time.

In this book, I will bring you on a journey of education and excitement to show you that walking is the tool that will deliver real and long-term transformation. As well as providing simple ways to improve your overall health, this book will transform your wellness with straightforward, actionable, experience-led tips and content that works.

The Walking Effect is my passion project. It is a book I have had in my mind for a long time and one I believe has the power to really change people's lives. I want you to use this book in a few ways.

1 To educate yourself on why we should walk. Don't worry, I'm not going to get too deep into the science, but I always think that being educated is the simplest way to motivate yourself. With some basic knowledge about the effects of walking on the body and mind, as well as information on how to make your walk more enjoyable, I know that you are more likely to walk more and make better choices more often. In the same way, when you know how to read food labels, you can make better choices about the food you eat; when you learn how to set goals properly, you stay motivated for life, not just for the short term.

2 As a guide book. In the second half of the book you will find some of my favourite walks in each province in Ireland. I really hope that some of these walks will take you to parts of Ireland you haven't been to before. Walking can bring you on an adventure and I hope the walks in this book will provide a bucket list for you! I post all my walks on my Instagram account and I hope these will further inspire you with new routes and new places to go.

3 As a kick-start. Maybe you haven't walked in twenty years and think you'd like to start. Maybe you want to walk 5km. Maybe you want to walk a marathon. Maybe you want to do more than just stroll each day and really get the benefits of walking as a form of exercise. Well, *The Walking Effect* can help you do all of these. Throughout the book, I'll show you just how easy it can be to make some simple changes and motivate you to take that very first step to health and wellness.

I hope this book will inspire you to get out and explore the world around you on your own two feet. It will be many things to many people, so read it and use it in whatever way suits you best.

I have seen just how powerful walking is and I believe that this book has the power to make positive changes in your life.

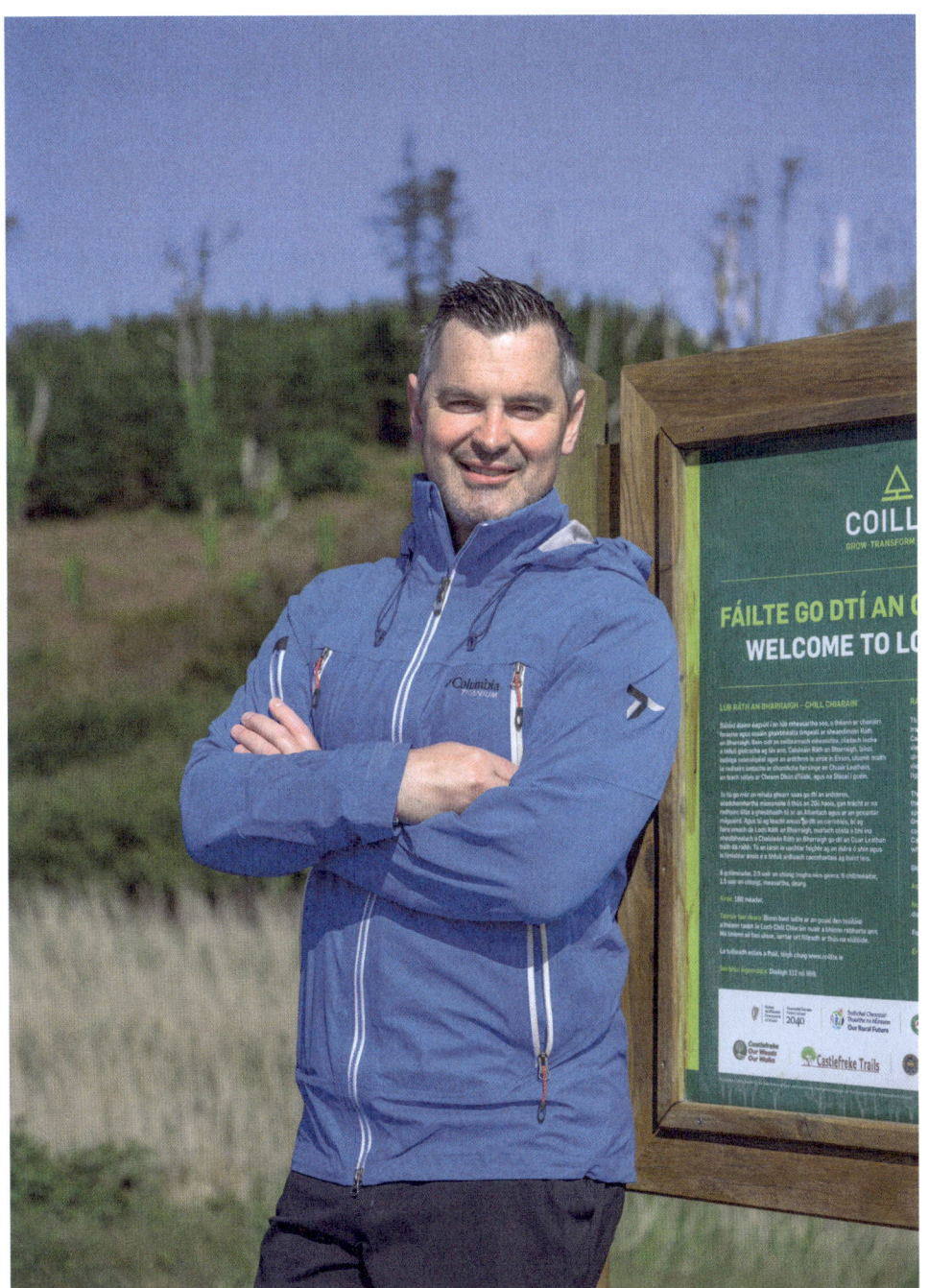

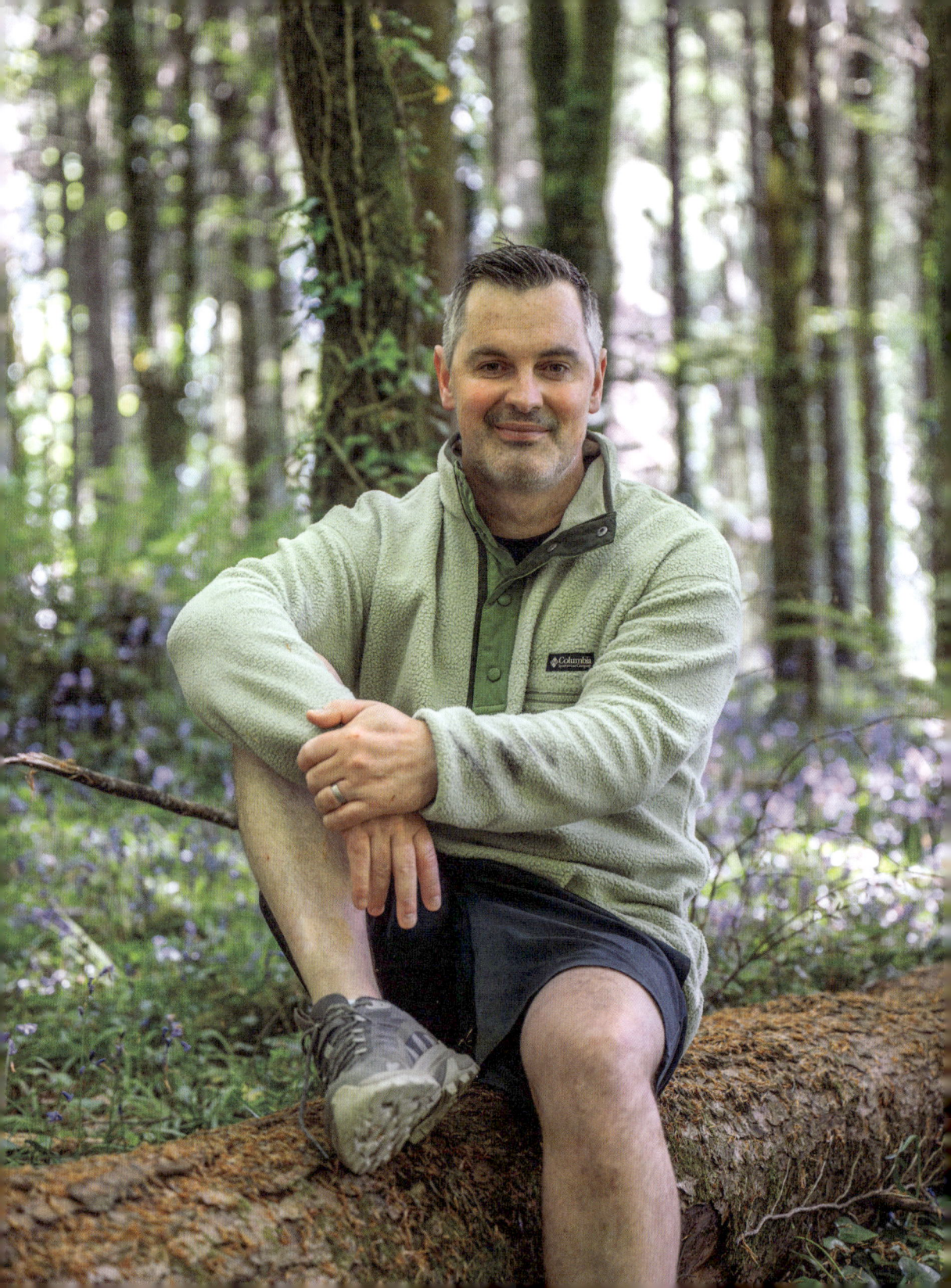

CHAPTER ONE

THE SCIENCE OF WALKING

MODERN LIFE IS INCREASINGLY SEDENTARY — NOW IS THE TIME TO WALK

As a society we are sitting more and more. The way we live is ageing us more quickly, making us weaker and increasing our anxiety. It is no surprise that all those problems are linked to the fact that we are moving less and less. Yes, a percentage of the population may go to the gym, but it is our general daily movement (GDM) that is reducing and that is the biggest issue of all.

I am always surprised when I see people taking the sedentary option when they are presented with a choice. I notice this all the time – people using the lift rather than the stairs or sitting at their desks all day, when they could be out walking in their lunch hour. I just wish people would take those first steps and feel the benefits. By choosing more opportunities to move, you will feel better and be healthier.

In a world of busyness and distractions, putting one foot in front of the other will help you to:

+ regulate your nervous system
+ deal with stress
+ live longer
+ live better
+ live stronger
+ work better
+ interact better
+ avoid falls
+ think better
+ feel less anxious

… and a whole lot more. As a society, moving less has made us anxious and burnt out. The fatigue of getting through a stressful, busy and sedentary day leaves us worried and empty, and I truly believe that our mental health has never been under more pressure.

Taking every opportunity to move can change that. Regularly choosing the stairs rather than the lift when you get to the office will deliver a shot of endorphins through your body, give you

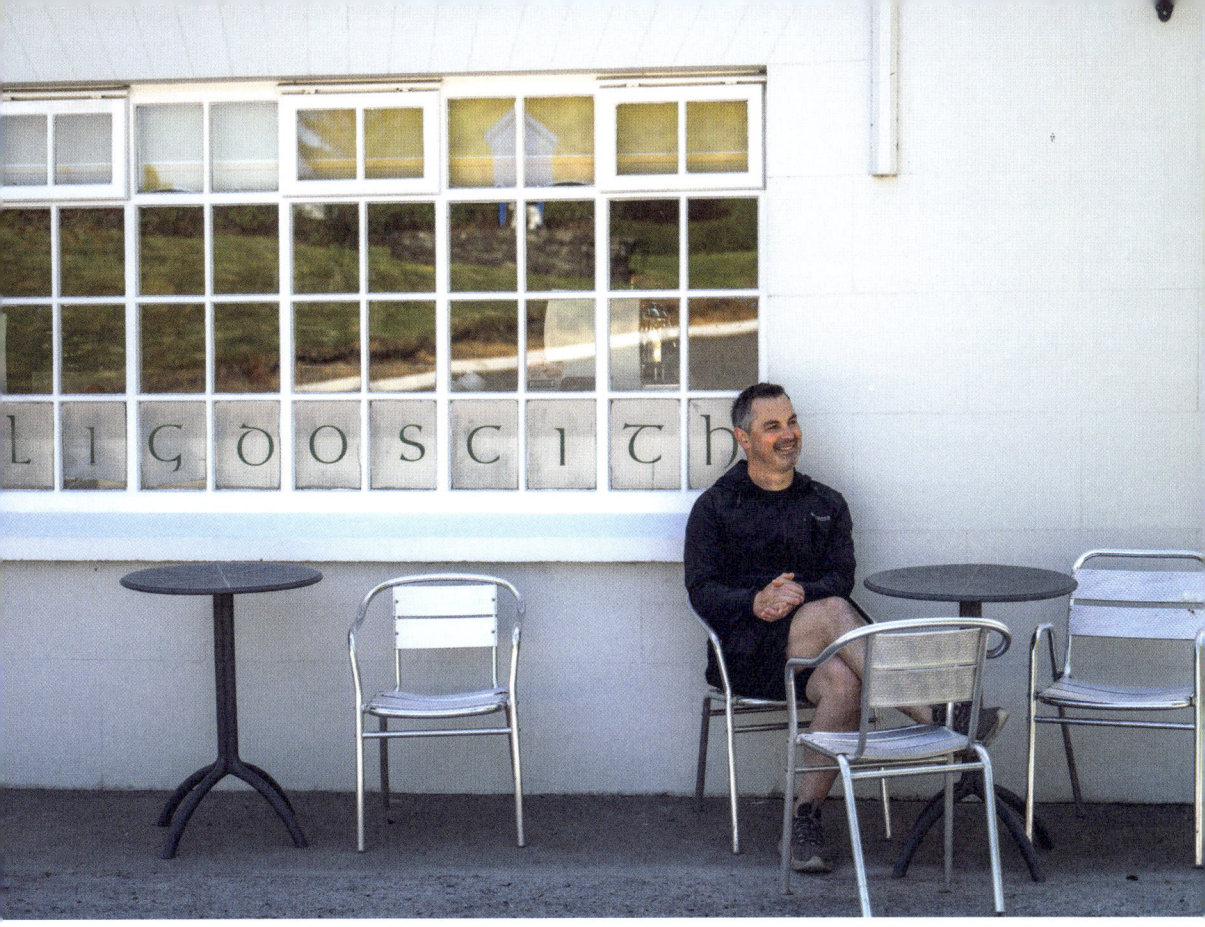

a surge of energy, reduce stress, build muscles in your legs, lower your resting heart rate, clear your brain fog, improve your core and lots more. Motivated yet?

Think about the last time you went to the supermarket or a shopping centre. Where did you park? I'd bet my house that you not only looked for the space closest to the door but that you also circled the car park trying to find that space when over on the other side of the car park, the area furthest away from the entrance, there were lots of spaces available. What this shows is the power of the subconscious mind – we are subconsciously seeking ease and ways of making our lives more sedentary. Increasing rates of osteoporosis, muscle atrophy (loss of muscle mass), balance-related falls, increased visceral fat (the fat that is stored around the tummy and surrounds our internal organs, and too much of which is dangerous for our health) and increased weight can all be attributed to how we are living. I am asking you to change that, and to use this book as a guide to help you live better and live longer.

The World Health Organization (WHO) monitors trends in physical inactivity. In a recent study it found that nearly one-third (31 per cent) of the world's adult population, 1.8 billion adults, are physically inactive. That is, they do not meet the global recommendations of at least 180 minutes of moderate-intensity physical activity per week. This is an increase of five percentage points between 2010 and 2022. If this trend continues, the proportion of adults not meeting recommended levels of physical activity is projected to rise to 35 per cent by 2030.

+ Globally, there are notable age and gender differences in levels of physical inactivity.
+ Women are less active than men by an average of five percentage points. This has not changed since 2000.
+ After 60 years of age physical inactivity levels increase in both men and women.
+ 81 per cent of adolescents (aged 11–17 years) were physically inactive.
+ Adolescent girls were less active than adolescent boys, with 85 per cent of girls (78 per cent of boys) not meeting WHO guidelines.

The WHO stats show you just how inactive we are becoming. The minimum recommendation is 180 minutes a week and nearly 30 per cent of people don't do that amount of movement.

You don't have to hike or take a brisk walk. Increasing your general daily movement can be as simple as parking further away from your workplace, the shops, school … Or you could choose to take the stairs instead of the lift. Do more housework. Leave the car at home and travel on foot.

I call these micro-choices. A micro-choice is a decision about a small but important daily task that can make a difference to your health. Walking is so often one of these micro-choices you can make. Micro-choices follow the 1 per cent rule, the idea that small changes add up to significant improvements over time. This is very much the principle outlined by James Clear in his book *Atomic Habits*. The idea is that the habits are so small that you barely notice them, so they don't feel like a big effort. The next time you are faced with a micro-choice, have a think about what you want to choose. Take that opportunity to move. These decisions, this attitude to life, are an expression of wanting to live better, be healthier, be stronger.

WHAT HAPPENS TO YOUR BODY WHEN YOU WALK?

People know that a walk will make them feel better, but what does it actually do? For your heart, your lungs, your mind, your muscles, your brain? Without getting too technical, I think it is really important not just to tell you that walking makes you feel better but to show you the science and how that science backs up what I am saying.

Walking is one of our most ancient physical functions. It is something we have always done and our bodies are adapted to do it. The body is an amazing machine – it adapts to the environment it is placed in. Apply that to our current environment, one of less movement and more sitting, and you will understand why our bodies are changing for the worse.

So let's take a look at what actually happens to our bodies when we walk and move. Walking doesn't just make us feel good; it does our bodies good too! Here's how.

Walking on a regular basis will:

+ Lower stress and tension
+ Improve your mood
+ Improve your cognitive health
+ Improve your balance and co-ordination
+ Improve your sleep
+ Make your bones stronger
+ Give you more energy
+ Strengthen your muscles
+ Reduce your body fat
+ Reduce the risk of health-related diseases, e.g. cardiovascular disease, stroke risk, etc.
+ Improve your core strength.

WHAT HAPPENS TO YOUR HEART WHEN YOU WALK?

Your heart is a muscle. It is the engine of the body. It pumps blood and oxygen around the body and delivers carbon dioxide to the lungs to be removed. Your heart is a muscle that can be trained to be healthier and pump more efficiently. When it gets stronger it pumps better.

Your resting heart rate is a good measure of your cardiovascular fitness and your stress levels too. It simply tells you how many times your heart has to beat each minute to keep you alive. The lower the number (for most people), the stronger your heart and the healthier you are. If you are going to take your resting heart rate, measure it in the morning before you have had any tea or coffee. For most people your resting heart rate should be between sixty and eighty beats per minute. Don't worry if your rate is lower than this; very fit people can often have a resting heart rate of forty to sixty beats per minute. If you are over-training or stressed, your resting heart rate will normally go up and this is a great signal to rest up and improve your overall health. If your resting heart rate is high I would always recommend going to see your GP. In a study about the effects of walking on risk factors for cardiovascular disease, Professor Elaine Murtagh and other experts found that:

> **Evidence from epidemiological studies suggests that even small improvements in the amount of daily walking is better than no walking, and greater increases confer larger cardiovascular health benefits. Patients may accrue short-terms gains such as improved fitness, body composition, blood pressure and lipid profiles. Longer-term benefits include reduced risk of CHD [coronary heart disease], coronary events and mortality. Patients should gradually raise their walking levels, with the [US] public health recommendation of 150 minutes per week as a minimum goal.**

When you walk, you are:

+ Increasing your heart rate and getting your heart to work harder, pump more and get stronger
+ Reducing the stress hormones that place extra pressure on your heart
+ Lowering your blood pressure
+ Lowering your cholesterol
+ Improving the health of your arteries
+ Helping to maintain a healthy weight.

WHAT HAPPENS TO YOUR LUNGS WHEN YOU WALK?

We all need oxygen to live and we get this from the air around us. The lungs' main job is to move fresh air into our body while removing waste gases.

When air comes into your lungs, oxygen is moved into the bloodstream and carried through your body. Your bloodstream then carries carbon dioxide back to the lungs, where it is removed from the bloodstream and exhaled.

When you walk or do any form of exercise, the body has to work harder and your lungs take in more air. As you walk more and get fitter, your muscles will become stronger and as a result need less oxygen and produce less carbon dioxide. In a nutshell, everything becomes more efficient. As reported by Asthma + Lung UK, 'Regular movement is good for your lungs because it increases the strength of the muscles around your lungs and the rest of your body. As you build strength, your muscles need less oxygen to work. This means you will be able to breathe more easily when you're active.'

There is more and more research telling us that nasal breathing (breathing in and out through your nose) when moving is a really easy way to increase the benefits we get from exercise. While it may feel odd at first, nasal breathing will help you and your lungs/heart benefit even more from the walk.

Simply try to walk with your mouth closed, slowly at first, then faster as you become more comfortable. You will find it harder to start with and all the muscles associated with breathing will tire a lot more quickly too, but as with everything, they will get stronger with practice and time. Sometimes people like to make this harder and tape their mouths during exercise, but I think this really isn't necessary – like everything else, this kind of breathing just takes practice.

WHAT HAPPENS TO YOUR MUSCLES AND BONES WHEN YOU WALK?

Our muscles and bones are what keep us strong and what help us to age better. The stronger they are, the less likely we are to trip or fall. We begin to lose muscle and bone strength in our thirties, and as the decades pass, the rate at which we lose that muscle and bone strength accelerates. This is especially true for women as they go through menopause and after. Over two in three women in Ireland over the age of 65 have osteoporosis, a condition that causes bones to become fragile and break more easily.

Bone health is so important. Having weak bones means it is more likely that a fall or trip will result in a fracture or a break. The good news is that you can strengthen your bones at any age through movement and eating better.

And we can slow and stabilise the process of muscle and bone strength loss by taking simple actions for our health. Standing and walking are two ways to do just that, and they help to strengthen everything.

Walking obviously uses all the muscles in the lower body, but it also engages your core muscles. Add in a backpack and you'll be working a host of upper-body muscles as well. Walking more will improve the strength of your muscles and help make your bones stronger, but here are a few additional simple ways to help your body even more:

+ Introduce 30-second bursts of speed to your usual walks. Simple but very effective.
+ Walk up and down hills.
+ Walk faster generally, or walk with someone faster than you.
+ Do some exercises during your walk, like press-ups on a bench or tricep dips.
+ Use a weighted vest or backpack.

A study by Krall and Hughes in the *American Journal of Medicine* found that:

> **Healthy postmenopausal women who walk approximately 1 mile each day have higher whole-body bone density than women who walk shorter distances. Walking is also effective in slowing the rate of bone loss from the legs.**

Isn't it incredible that just one mile a day, which for most people is a 15–20 minute walk, can deliver such great results? And it's free!

WHAT HAPPENS TO YOUR MIND WHEN YOU WALK?

When you walk, there is an increased flow of blood, oxygen and nutrients to your brain. A protein called brain-derived neurotrophic factor (BDNF) is also released. This stimulates the growth of new brain cells and connections, which helps your brain to work better and improves your memory.

In a trial with 120 people aged 55 to 80, researchers at the University of Illinois compared the effects of walking for 40 minutes three times a week with the effects of stretching exercises. Over a year, the part of the brain responsible for memory, the hippocampus, decreased in size by 1 per cent in the stretching group but increased by 2 per cent in the walking group. Two per cent!

Walking is nature's way to clear the head, relax the mind and help you to focus better. Even taking a few minutes outside – parking further away and walking to your meeting, or doing the school pick-up on foot – can make a big difference. It all comes down to making the right choice by taking as many opportunities to move as you can throughout your day, your week, your month and your year.

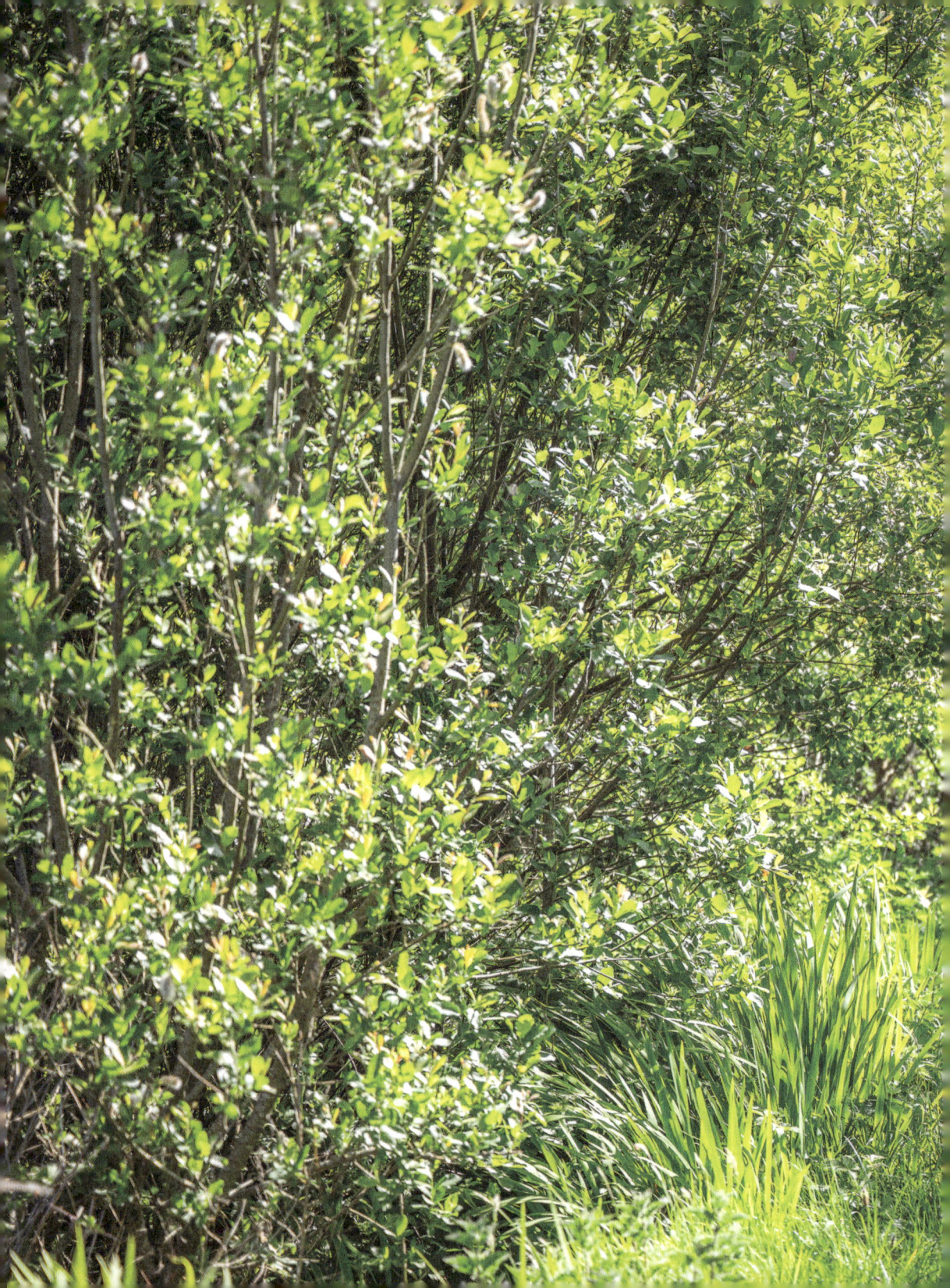

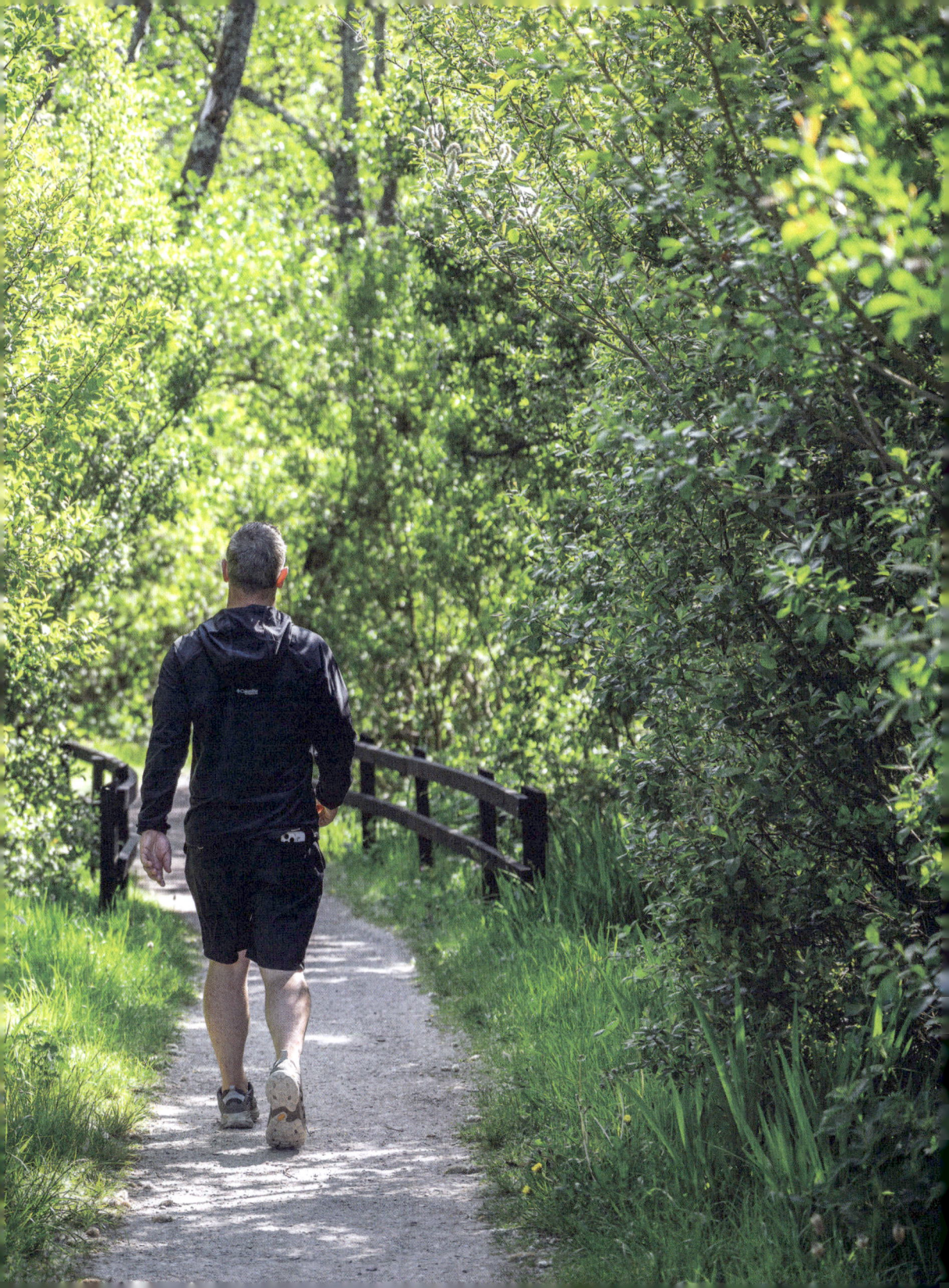

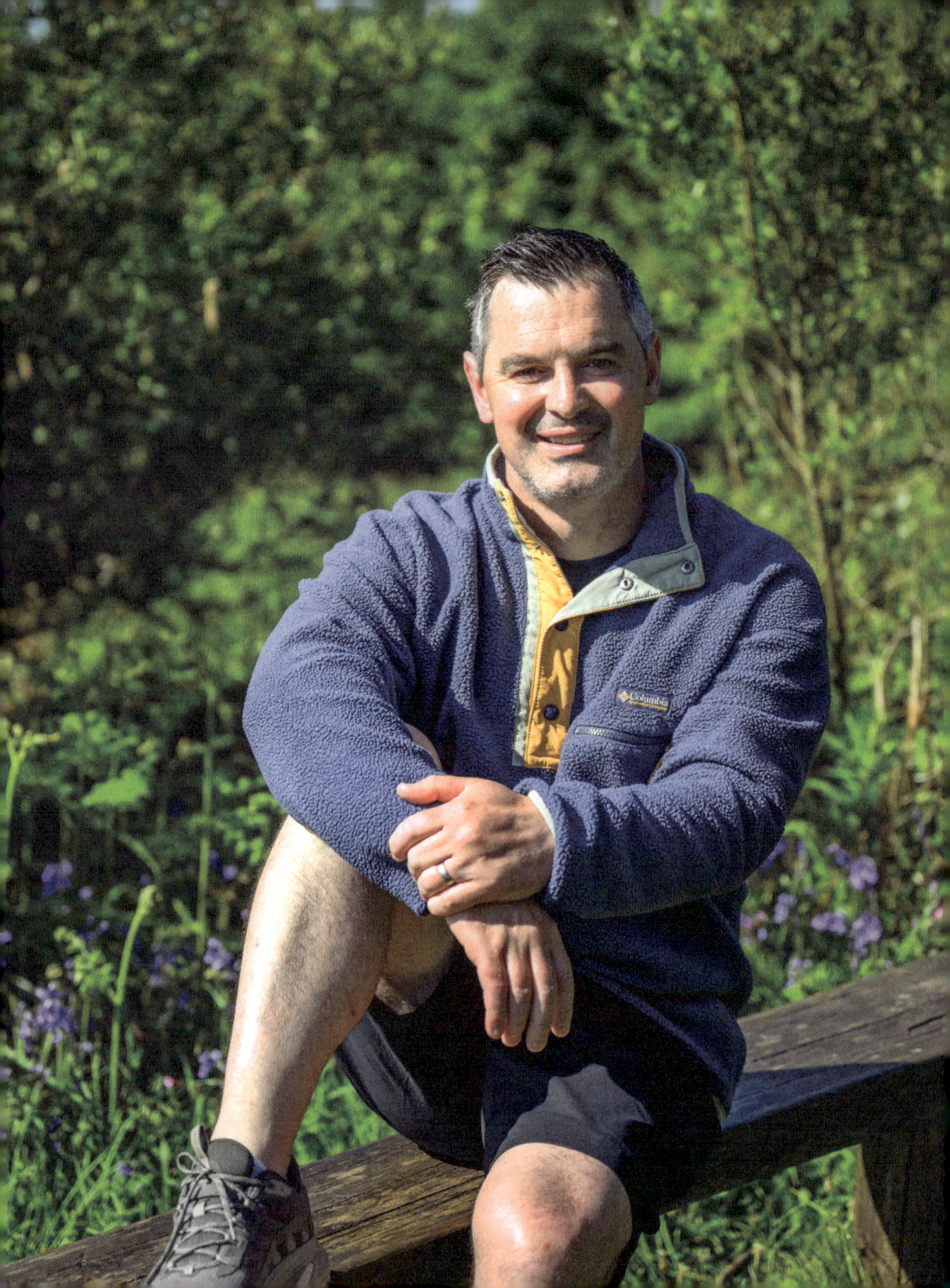

CHAPTER TWO

HOW TO WALK BETTER

In the previous chapter, we looked at why walking is such great exercise and what it can do for you. Now I want to give you some simple tips to help you walk better and enable you to get more out of it. Let's take a look at how some easy changes can make your walking even better.

GETTING GOING

Do you know what the hardest part of any walk is? The first 30 seconds. If you feel overwhelmed by the thought of walking, focus on the start. Get your shoes on and just do 30 seconds. I know that feeling myself, and guess what? I have never turned back after 30 seconds. Ever. Just get yourself out the door, or to the end of the driveway, or onto the greenway, or along the first side of the pitch while you're watching your child at training. You will keep going because you have done the hard work – getting started!

WALKING TECHNIQUE

Now, I know what you're thinking. Surely you can just walk? Yes, of course you can, but there are some simple ways to do it better. This is especially true when you start walking faster, or if you are just starting out and haven't walked any sort of distance for a long time. Fast walking delivers even more benefits to your health, but when your stride starts to lengthen and your pace increases, your technique becomes more important too!

Your posture, core and eyeline can really make a big difference to your walk and the impact it has on your body. Now, it is important to remember that everyone walks differently and we all move differently. There's so much pressure placed on people to be perfect – to have the perfect posture, the perfect gait, the perfect flexibility – but I tend to shy away from that. I think we should all work to the best of our ability, to how we are mechanically made, and just do our best. If your technique isn't 100 per cent perfect, that's perfectly fine in my opinion. The most important thing is to get moving!

With all this in mind, I still want to describe the ideal way your body should look when you're walking, so that you have something to aim for, and so that you can keep it in mind when you're on the move.

+ Your head is up. You're looking forward, not down at the ground. When most of us walk, we tend to look down. This is especially true when we have a phone in our hand. Scrolling while walking fast is a recipe for a sore neck and sore shoulders! Your eyeline should be straight ahead, so you can still see the ground in case there are any trips or hazards in front of you. This instantly improves your posture, reduces your neck and shoulder tension, and relaxes your upper body. If this seems too scary, adjust your eyeline gradually over time. Adjusting your eyeline comes down to confidence: as you begin to become more confident in your stride and your strength, you will become more comfortable looking further ahead. This adjustment will also help you to lift your feet a little further off the ground if, like me, you have a tendency to drag your feet. Making a conscious effort to lift your feet will feel strange initially but it will make your walk a lot safer and help prevent trips and falls.

+ Your neck, shoulders and back are relaxed, not stiffly upright or tense. If you find you are carrying tension in your neck and shoulders, try some of the stretches later in the book and make a conscious effort to relax when walking. The gradient of your walk can make a big difference with this – walks with hills will impact far more on your upper body – so if you are starting out, a flat walk will be much more suitable and comfortable for you.

+ *Arms:* Ideally, you are swinging your arms freely with a slight bend in your elbows. Sometimes people find that their hands tend to swell when they are walking, but bringing your hands higher than your elbows every few minutes will help to improve the circulation in your hands and make them so much more comfortable. When you are really walking fast, using your arms to help drive your stride length and up the pace can make a big difference. Sometimes you will see people using hand weights to make this movement a little harder – adding weights can force your arms to work a little harder and strengthen them too.

+ *Core:* While you are walking, pull your belly button in towards your spine to engage your core. Your back is straight, not arched forwards or backwards; you are tall and proud. Our core muscles are put to work with pretty much every daily task that we do. You can strengthen your core by just moving more and moving a little harder. Adding the exercises in this book or from my Instagram into your day will make a big difference too. Just remember that sit-ups don't give you a flatter stomach or necessarily a stronger core, though people often think that they do. Full body movements will do a whole lot more!

+ *Stride:* When you are walking, for most people, you are walking with a heel strike, walking heel to toe and really pushing off the front of the foot. This is why checking your gait is so important when buying your runners. How your foot hits the ground dictates everything.

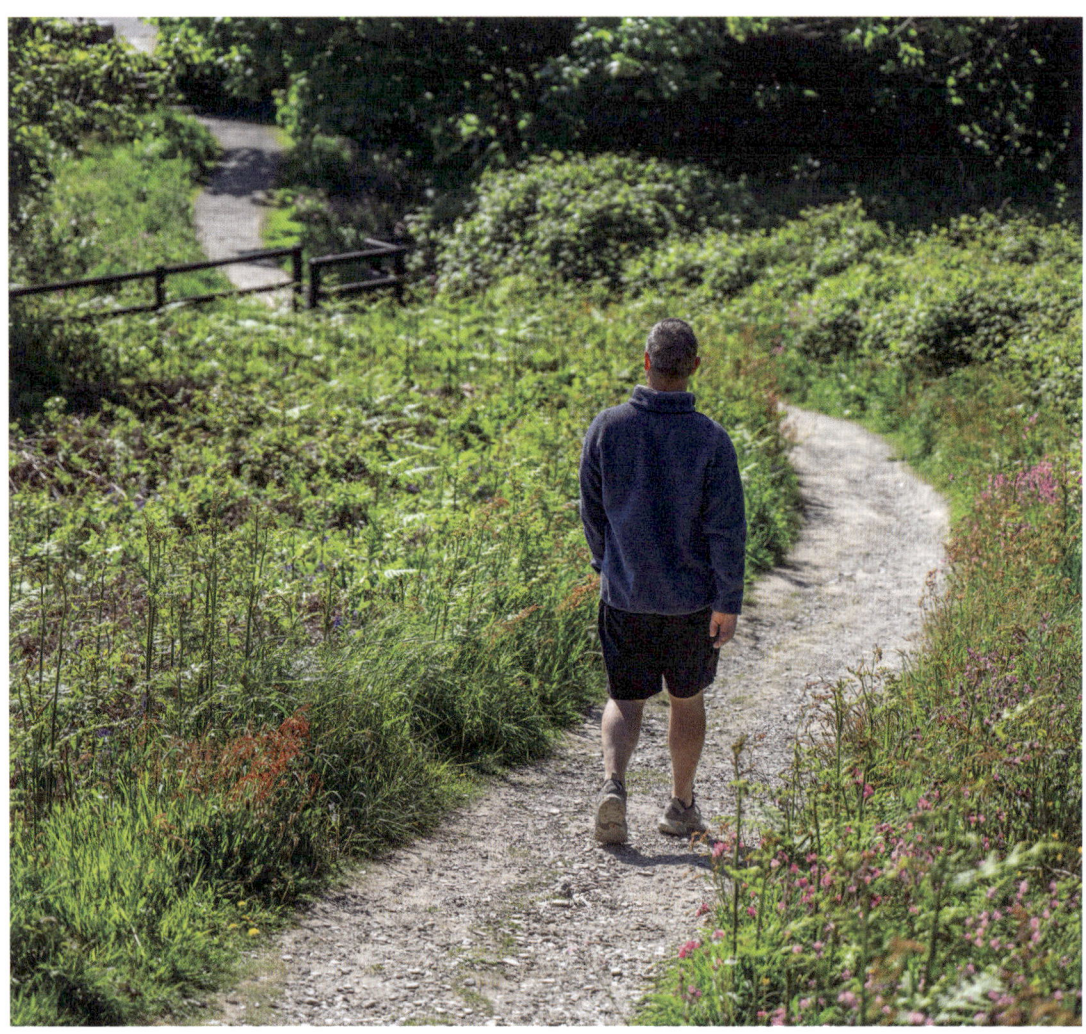

TYPES OF WALKING

Let's take a look at the different types of walking and what each one can do for you. Not all walking is the same – each kind can deliver different benefits.

STROLLING

Strolling is just general movement, for example walking around the office, around the house, just moving during the day without really thinking about it. It is your 10,000-steps-a-day kind of movement. Really low intensity, never out of breath and often just unconsciously doing it. It is great for getting the body out and about and it does provide some benefits, but it isn't exercise. It isn't challenging the body hard enough to deliver real exercise benefits for most people. But if you haven't moved for a long time, this can be a great place to start!

WALKING

Next up the intensity ladder is actual walking when you're out of the house. You're taking the pace up a notch, you have a longer stride and you're starting to get some of the hormonal benefits of stress release and challenging your body enough to change. Your core and waist are working harder and you're breathing a little faster. Another great form of movement, it is exercise – and exercise you can do when you're going to work or wherever.

FAST WALKING

Now you are really exercising and pushing the pace. Fast walking is one of the best exercises you can do. It's great for your lungs, your core, your back and a whole lot more – and it's free. People often ask me how they'll know if they are walking fast enough. The answer is that you can tell you have achieved this pace when you are huffing and puffing, feeling challenged and as though you've had a workout when you're done.

HILLWALKING

Now you take advantage of your fitness levels to explore and experience some adventure. Ireland is an incredible country for hillwalking. Have a look at some of the suggested walks later in the book and try them for yourself. Brilliant for the legs, hips, bum and core, there is nothing that hillwalking doesn't benefit. It tends to be longer in duration, so planning and preparing is important, as well as health and safety.

WALKING INDOORS

Guess what? Those steps you take around the house when you are doing housework are a fantastic form of movement and exercise. Lifting, hoovering and going up and down the stairs are things we need to keep doing for as long as possible, especially as we get older.

Walking pads and treadmills are also great ways to walk indoors. Walking pads have become really trendy of late. Put simply, they are cheap and basic treadmills. They are small and portable, and provide a great way to help people just move at home.

The next step up is a treadmill, which is more expensive. It's sturdy and has an incline, along with programmes to follow, so a treadmill is a great investment if you find you want to move on from a walking pad or have joint or weight considerations. They have better suspension and if you get a commercial one you will be using a machine that will make you want to keep using it.

I think there has been a huge increase in people who just don't feel comfortable walking outside or who feel self-conscious. We are becoming more and more aware of what other people think (or what we think they think). Walking indoors provides a safe space, and a space that can really help to improve our health and wellness.

RUCKING

In its simplest form, rucking is a way to make your walk harder by adding weight in a backpack or using a weighted vest on your shoulders. The principle here is pretty straightforward. As you get fitter and stronger, the walk becomes easier and the results or improvements begin to level off. Adding a bag or weighted vest makes your body adapt and strengthen as you are walking.

Getting fitted for the right backpack is important. The clips at chest height and waist height spread the weight of the backpack evenly across your body and can make a big difference to the comfort of the walk.

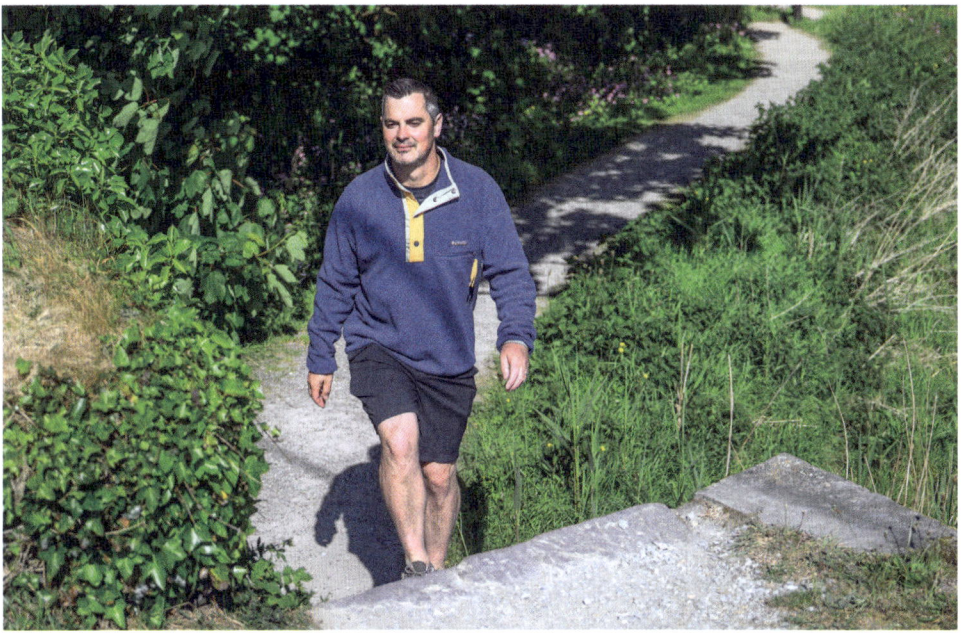

SIMPLE WAYS TO INCREASE YOUR WALKING PACE

You will know by now that I am always saying that fast walking is the ultimate exercise, and I always encourage my clients to push the pace. One of the first things people typically do when they try to walk faster is to take longer strides. Surprisingly, sometimes that tactic slows you down because it's harder to transfer your body weight to a foot that's too far in front of you if you make that stride too long.

The tips below will work for some people and variations of them will work for others. We all walk differently – it is so important to remember that! Try some of these suggestions and see how they make your walk feel. If you are tracking your walk you will be able to see what tips are working for you and what tips aren't in terms of pace and speed.

STAND TALL

Posture is so important, especially when you want to up the pace. Extend your spine as if you were being lifted by the crown of your head. When your posture is good and your core muscles are activated, you have a more powerful stride and feel more in control of your body when the going gets tough. Standing tall will also help alleviate aches and pains in your upper and lower back and allow you to take deep breaths for more energy as the muscles around your ribcage relax.

BEND YOUR ARMS

We have all seen people power-walking with their arms straight, looking as though they're flying along, but there is a better way to do it. You wouldn't run with your arms straight – it would slow you down and feel awkward. The same goes for walking. When you bend your arms, it's easier to swing them fast. And since your body likes to be in sync, your legs will speed up to stay in time with your arms. Bend your elbows 85° to 90° and swing your arms forward and back—not side to side or diagonally across your body. The added momentum of using your arms really helps you to walk faster.

LAND ON YOUR HEEL

There are two ways your foot should strike the ground when you are walking. Heel to toe is the most common; a mid-point foot strike is another. For a lot of people, landing on your heel and rolling through your foot is one of the ways to help you power on. As your leg swings forward, your heel should be the first part of your foot that makes contact with the ground. Focus on keeping your toes up as you land. This facilitates the heel-to-toe walking motion that will make it easier to walk faster than if your foot slaps down on the ground with each step. Roll from your heel to your toes as smoothly as possible. Finally, push off with your toes to propel you forward.

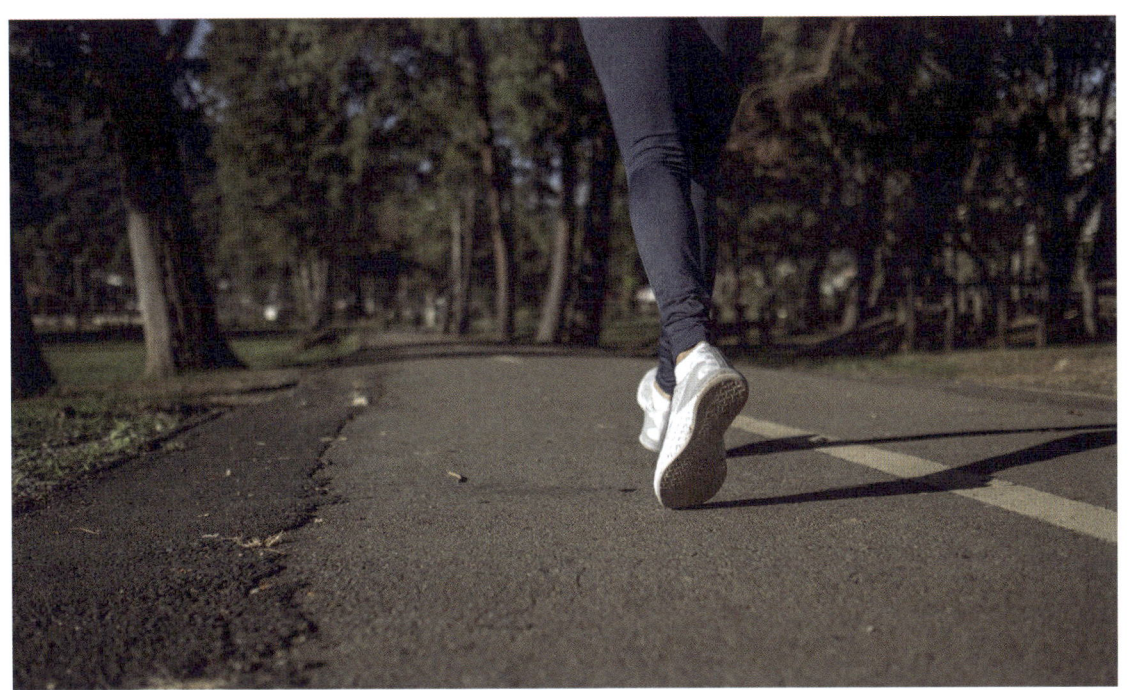

PUSH OFF STRONGLY

Focus on really pushing off the ground to propel yourself forward when you are starting into your next step. For maximum power, bend at the ball of your foot, raising your heel as if you were trying to show the person behind you the sole of your shoe.

TAKE SHORTER, QUICKER STEPS

People often reach a point where they can't make their stride any longer. This is a way to fix that, and it stops you over-striding (taking longer steps than normal). Instead, focus on shorter, quicker steps – place your front leg almost directly under you as you fall into your next step. This allows for a smoother, rolling stride that makes it easier for you to shift your body weight to your front leg, then swing your back leg forward. The result: a faster walking speed.

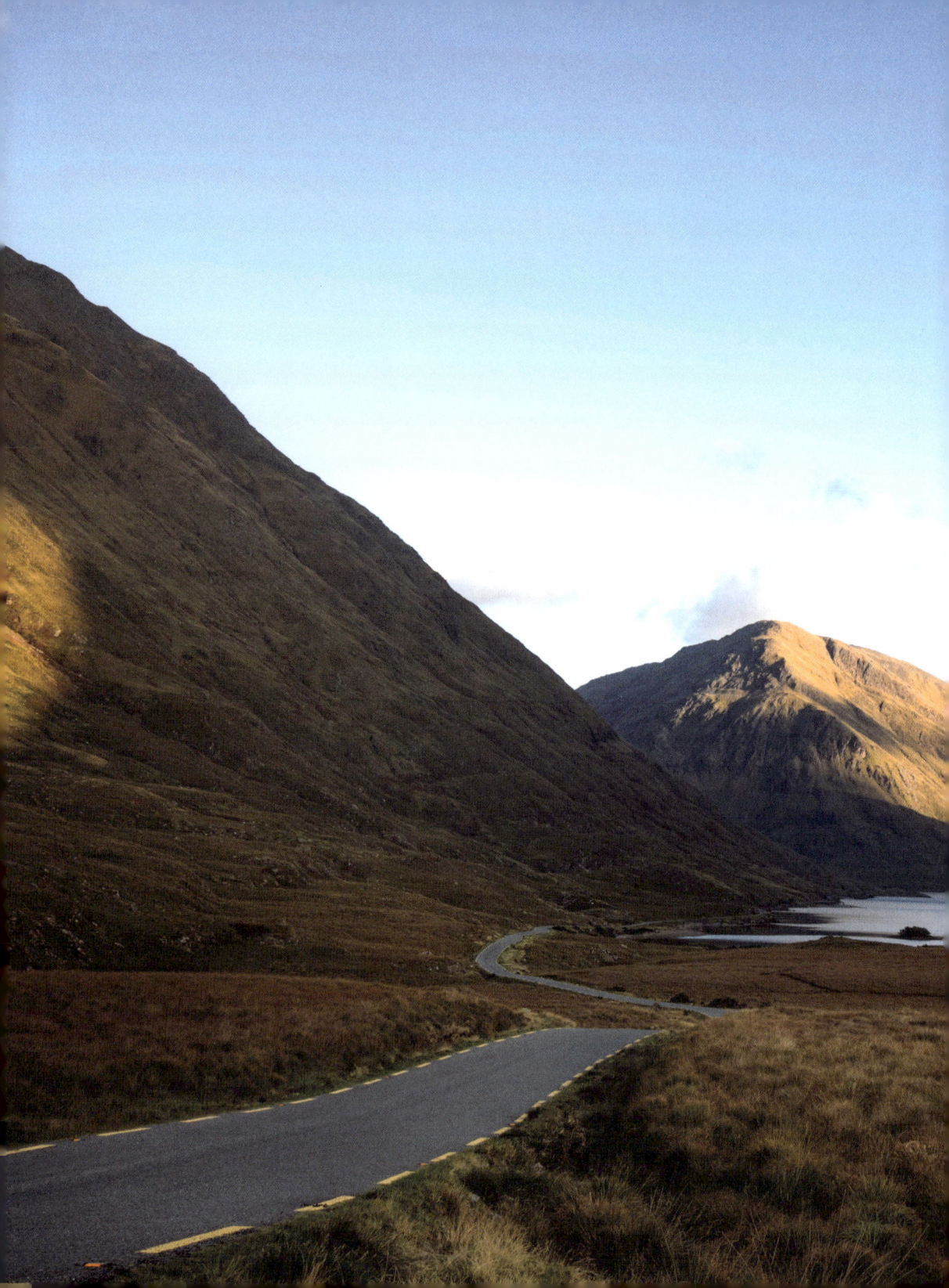

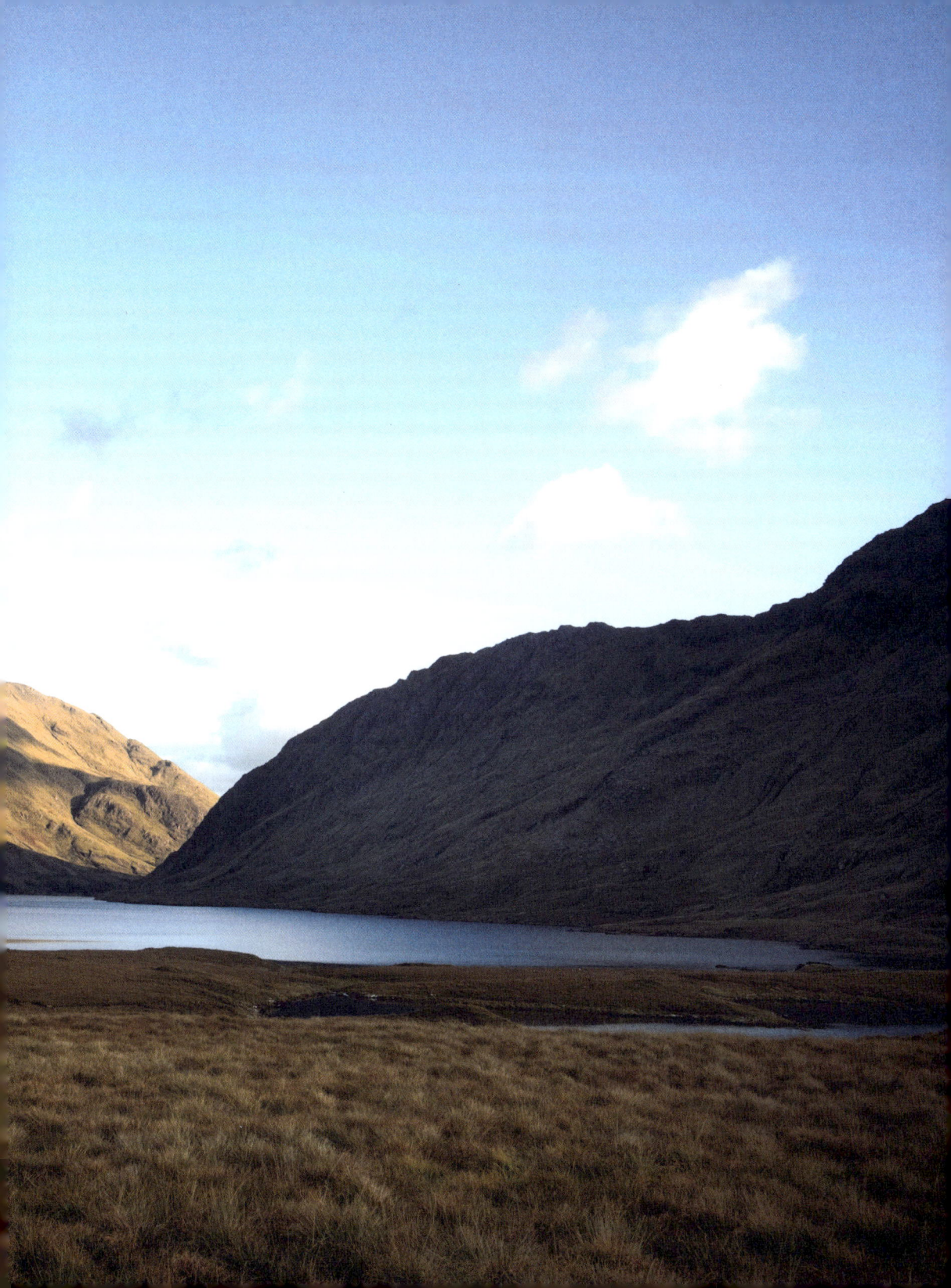

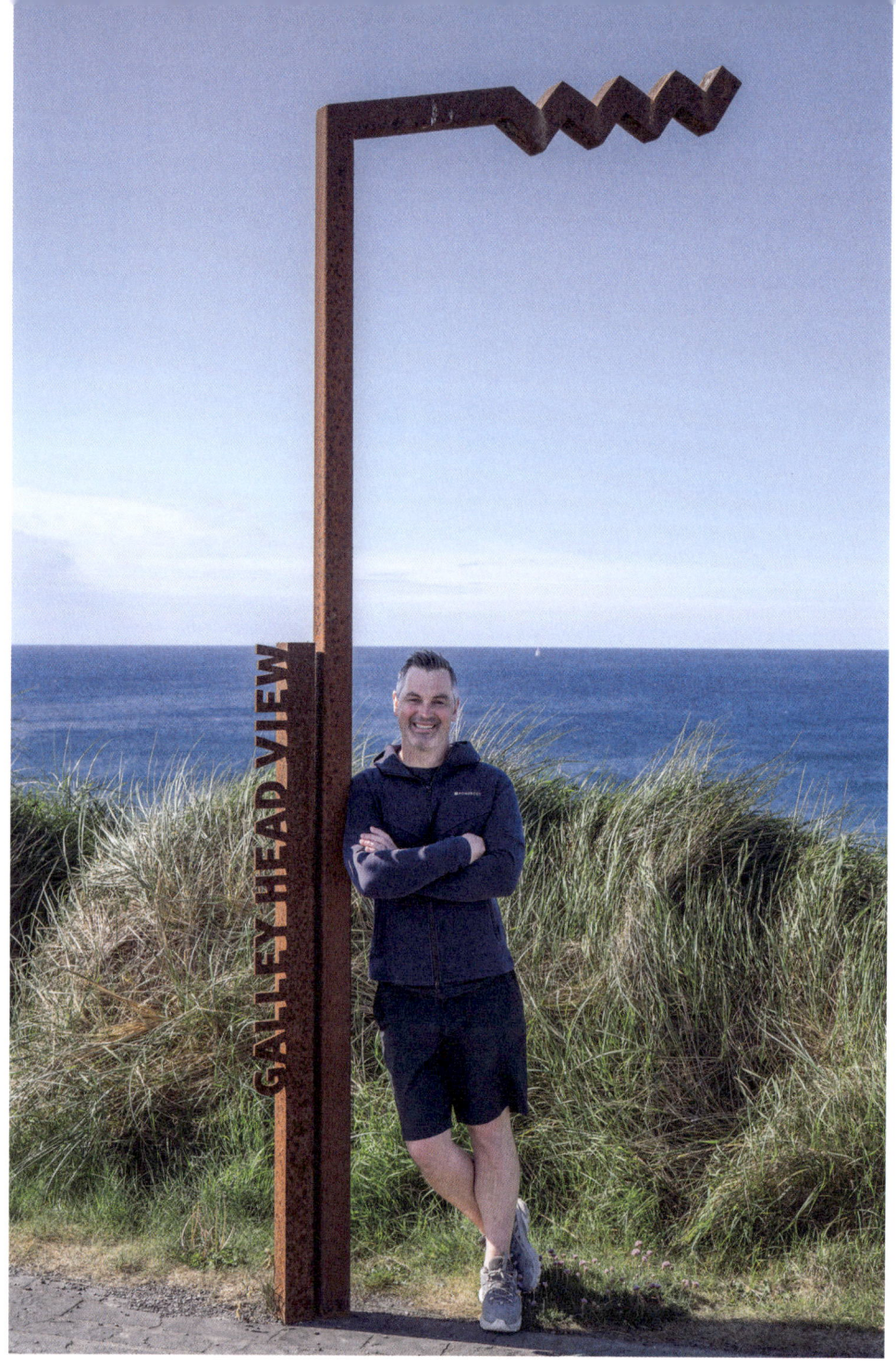

USING YOUR BREATH

Breathing is something we do without even thinking about it. Yet by learning to breathe properly, you can dramatically improve your health. Simple adjustments will yield big results!

Robert J. Snyder, a respiratory therapist at University Hospitals, says:

> Certain breathing techniques have been proven to enhance the functioning of the heart and lungs, improve mental wellness, increase energy and concentration, and promote better sleep.

When deep breathing techniques are practised regularly and correctly, they can provide the following health benefits:

+ Lower blood pressure and heart rate. When you take deep, measured breaths, it triggers a relaxation response. Blood vessels open wider, making it easier for the heart to pump blood.
+ Reduced stress and anxiety. Slow, deliberate breathing sends a message to your brain that everything is okay. This calms the nervous system and reduces the level of stress hormones in the blood.
+ Enhanced immune response. Improved blood flow and lower levels of stress hormones help the body clear germs and viruses from the blood more efficiently.
+ Improved muscle function. The better blood flow that comes with relaxation delivers more oxygen and essential nutrients to the muscles so that they can function properly.

Here are some different ways to breathe that you can try on your next walk:

+ Pursed-lip breathing: Inhale deeply through your nose and exhale very slowly through pursed lips, with each exhalation lasting longer than the inhalation.
+ Diaphragmatic (belly) breathing: Place one hand on your chest and the other on your belly. Inhale deeply through your nose so that you can feel your belly expanding while your chest remains still. Then exhale slowly through your mouth.

+ 4–7–8 breathing: Breathe in for four seconds, hold your breath for seven seconds and then exhale through your mouth for eight seconds. This breathing exercise is known for its calming effects on the body and mind and may help some people fall asleep. When you're out for a slow de-stressing walk, it will really help you to calm and relax.

+ Alternate-nostril breathing: Use your ring finger to press one nostril closed. Keep your mouth closed and breathe in slowly through the open nostril. Release your finger and press the other nostril closed, while slowly and completely exhaling through the open nostril.

+ One-minute or box breath: Try this when you're going on one of those relaxing walks. Start walking and then take a deep breath in for five seconds, hold that breath for five seconds and then exhale gently and slowly for ten seconds. You can start with a shorter amount of time and work your way up to longer times, as long as the inhale and hold are the same length and the exhale is twice as long.

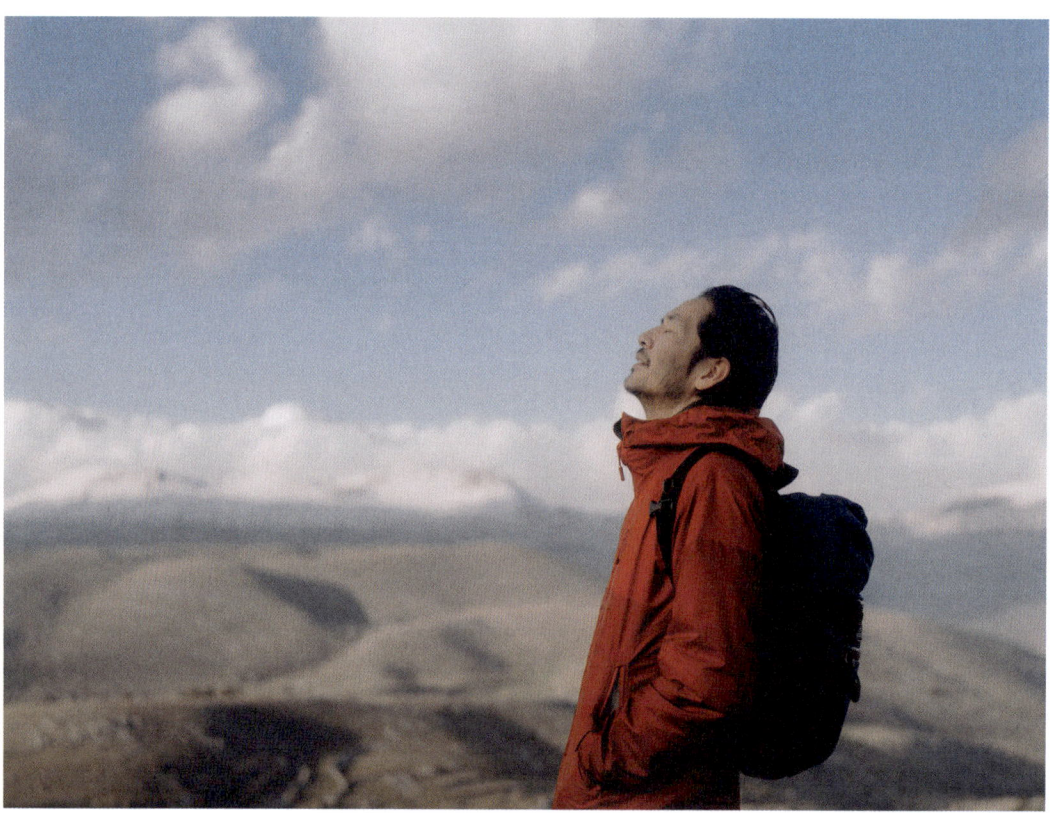

EXERCISES TO HELP YOU WALK BETTER

Walking on its own will make such a difference to your life. I hope you have seen that from the book so far. But adding some resistance exercises into your week will transform everything! People often get scared when we talk about resistance exercise or getting stronger. Don't be. These are simply exercises using your body weight or adding a set of dumbbells. They are simple exercises that you can do at home or in a gym to help you to stay strong.

If you do decide to make the leap and begin these exercises, ease yourself in gently. Try one set of the exercises, 15 repetitions, with plenty of breaks in between. As you get fitter and stronger you can build up to two or three sets with shorter rest times.

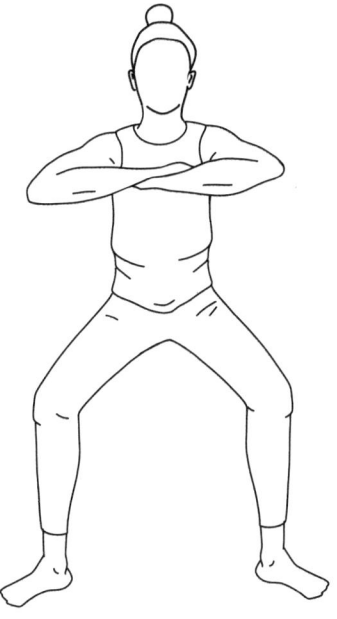

WIDE FOOT SQUATS

This is one of my favourite exercises for the legs. It's super for the insides of your legs, that soft part, and the outside of your bum, the part that you always want to lift.

Start the exercise with your feet wider apart than your shoulders, the wider the better. Turn your feet away from your body and lower your bum towards the floor and hold it there. This is your starting position. From there simply lower your bum towards the floor and pulse it around three inches. It's this pulsing motion that is doing all the toning.

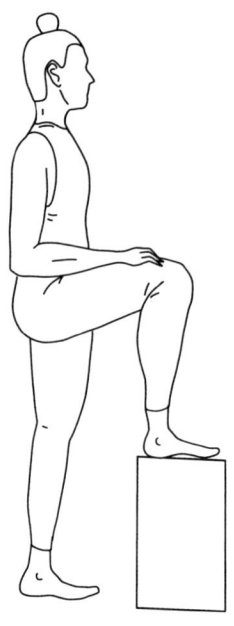

STEP-UPS

These are for the fit person only if using a higher bench, or you can start on a lower step. No matter how you do it, they are fantastic for toning the bum and the legs, and they're good for the aerobic system.

Stand in front of a park bench or a solid chair and ensure your back is straight. Place your hands on your hips, then step up with your right leg and back down. Repeat 15 times with the right leg and then switch to 15 with the left leg. Keep your hands on your hips and ensure your posture is good, especially towards the end of the set when the legs get tired. Fifteen might be a little too much at first, so just see how many you feel comfortable with and build it up as you get fitter and stronger.

PELVIC FLOOR KICKS

This is another simple exercise that is incredibly effective for the bum area and lifting the bum.

Start by lying on the floor on your back, with your knees bent, hands by your side. Now just push your pelvis towards the ceiling using all the muscles in your bum, return to the floor and push back up to the ceiling. If you find that it's too easy for you, just bring your heels closer to your body. If it's still too easy, hold for 30 seconds between sets.

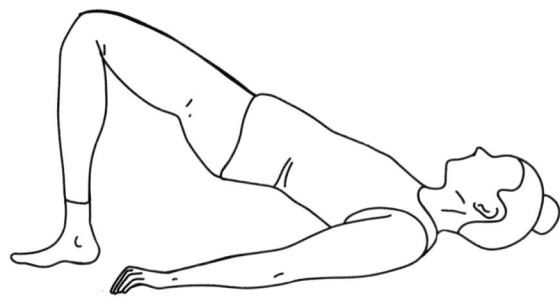

BRIDGE/PLANK

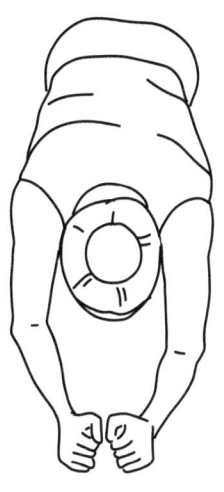

This is a classic exercise for the stomach and the centre core of the body. However, if you have back pain this is best avoided unless you have a fitness professional close by.

Start with your elbows on the floor and your toes on the floor, knees bent. Hold for 30 seconds and then release back down with your knees on the floor. This is the beginner's exercise, so if you want to advance it from here start by lifting your knees off the floor, keeping your back straight, and pull your belly button in towards your spine.

BICEP CURLS

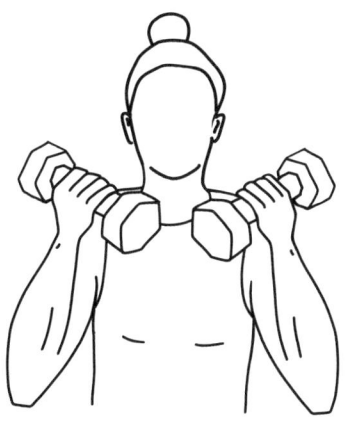

The old-school bicep exercise for the front of your arm, the curl is so easy to do. The important thing is to keep your elbows by your side and keep your back straight.

Simply raise the weight all the way up and all the way down.

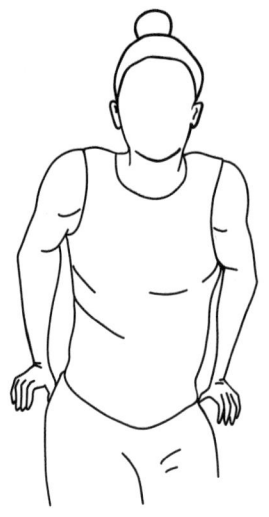

TRICEPS

Dips, dips and more dips! You've got to love these.

Start by sitting on a bench or a chair. Place your hands by your side and simply bend your elbows and, coming away from the chair, lower your body towards the floor and then extend your arms out. To make the exercise harder you can move your feet further away, but aim to keep your back beside the chair.

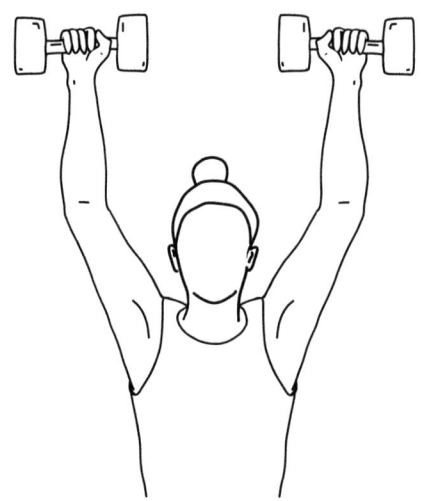

MILITARY PRESS

A simple yet effective shoulder exercise.

Get a couple of weights or water bottles and hold one in each hand. Start with your feet shoulder width apart, hands at your waist. Now bring the weights up to your shoulders, extend to the ceiling and then back to your shoulders, remembering not to arch your back. You can also do this exercise without the weights.

FRONT RAISE

A great exercise for your shoulders and your posture.

Start with your feet shoulder-width apart, back straight and arms extended in front of you with weights in your hands. Keeping your arms straight, simply raise your arms until they are at eye level.

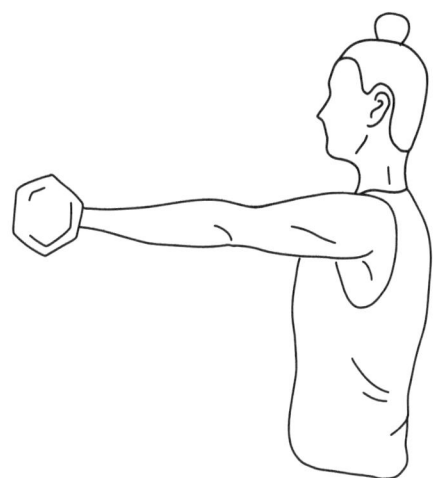

HOLDING SIT-UP

Simply lie on your back, hands by your sides and knees bent. Now raise your bum so that the quads at the front of your legs are parallel to the floor. Hold for as long as possible, keeping your back pushed towards the floor, especially as you get tired. If you have any back pain, stop straight away.

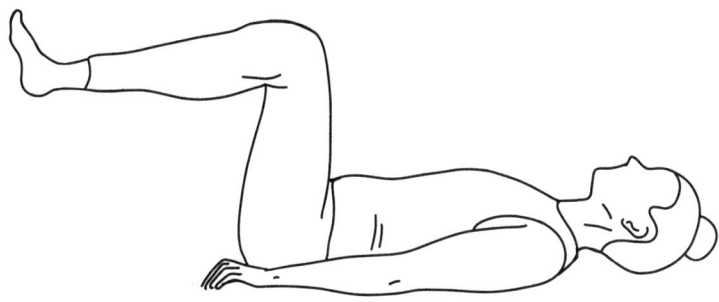

BUM KICKS

If you want a firmer, more toned bum you will want to do lots of these. Your glutes – your bum muscles – are so important for your balance and your strength.

Start on the floor on your hands and knees. Simply bring one knee into your chest, then extend your leg back towards the wall behind you. Repeat on the same leg 15 times and then do the same with the other leg. Aim to keep your back flat and ensure you kick your leg back until it's parallel to the floor.

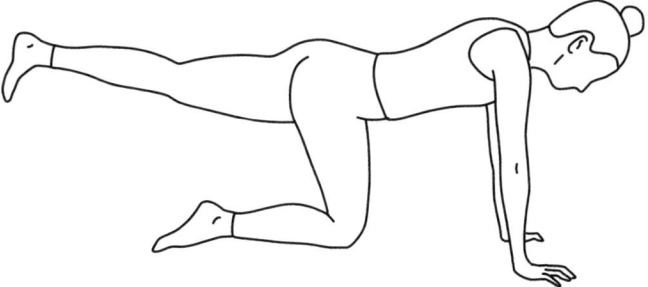

BACK LUNGES

Start with your feet together, standing tall and facing a wall or a chair for balance. Now step backwards with your right leg, bending your right knee towards the floor, and return to standing. It is essential to ensure that your back is straight all the way through the exercise, as when you get tired it will naturally want to bend. Do 15 reps on the right leg and then switch to the left leg for 15. Take a break for 30 seconds afterwards and then do a second and third set if you are able. The lower the leg goes towards the floor, the harder the exercise gets, so you can adjust it as feels comfortable for you.

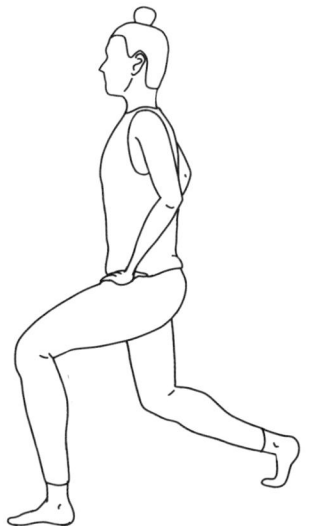

LYING CROSSOVERS

These are a great exercise for the stomach and pelvis region. If you have any back pain stop straight away.

Start by lying on your back on a mat or a towel. Place your hands under your lower back – this helps to support the back. Start with your legs straight. Simply cross your legs over and back, alternating the leg you lead with. The lower the legs go, the harder it will be, so just be careful with these and adjust according to how you feel.

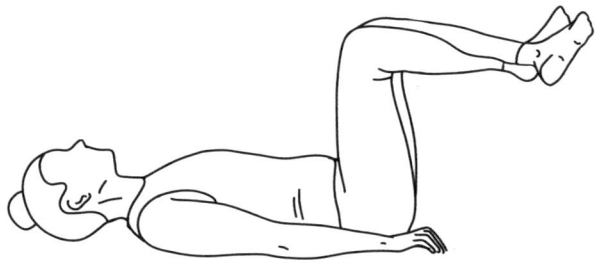

STRAIGHT ARM PLANK

A simple but great exercise for the middle part of the body.

Start on the floor, lying on your front, with your hands palms-down on the floor, shoulder-width apart, and your feet together. Now raise your body off the floor with your arms straight into a press-up position. Hold that position for as long as you can. Aim to start with 30 seconds and then build it up. Make sure you pull your stomach in towards your spine while holding, and keep your back straight.

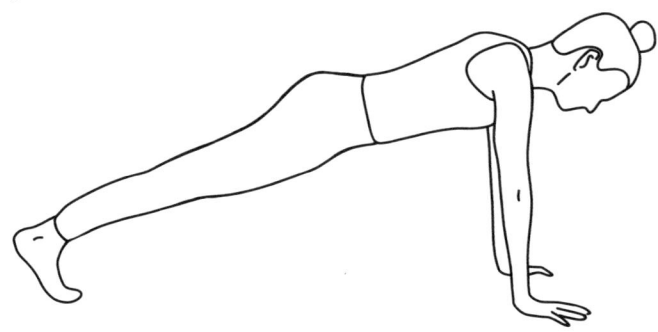

LET'S SET SOME GOALS

I hope some readers will buy this book to discover new hikes and that, for others, it will help to create a healthier lifestyle. Whatever your reason for buying *The Walking Effect*, thank you! And whatever your reason, I'd like to encourage you to set some goals and help you to achieve them. Setting a goal means that you have something to work towards. It means that you are far more likely to get there than by just hoping it might happen.

First, let me ask you a question. Why do you want to use walking to get healthier? And don't just give a quick throwaway answer, really think about it. Maybe apply the five-whys principle. Give five answers and then ask yourself 'Why?' for each answer you give. Then you will generally get to the real reason. It is a great way to delve into your mindset around your goals and it really works. For example: Why do you want to get fitter?

1   Why? To feel better.
2   Why? Because I feel tired all the time.
3   Why? Because that impacts how I feel in work and at home.
4   Why? Because it impacts my mood.
5   Why? I know feeling better will help me to live better and happier.

By doing a little bit of work on finding the right 'Why?', you are giving yourself the best chance of staying healthy for the long term. This is because you will have found a true reason, a deep meaningful reason to make those changes, to lace up those shoes, to put one foot in front of the other. When it means something to you, it matters, and that will be the driver behind you.

So get a cup of tea and pen and paper and sit down and work through your whys. You may be surprised by what you write down!

HOW TO STAY MOTIVATED ALL YEAR ROUND

Finding that 'Why?' is such a big step, so well done! It is often the hardest part that no one really does, but now that you have, let's take a look at some other really simple measures to help you stay motivated all year round.

VISION BOARD

A vision board is something I use myself. Each year I like to push my own boundaries of health and do something that pushes me physically and scares me psychologically. This year, for example, I am swimming to the Fastnet lighthouse and back to Baltimore in the summer (I love lighthouses) and I'm going to swim the length of Loch Ness in Scotland (I am also fascinated by the Loch Ness monster). So to help myself stay motivated, I have one poster of each in the gym and my office. I see them several times each day. On the days I don't want to train, having them there makes me want to go. They are both vision boards.

It might be a picture of that holiday destination you are going to, that item of clothing you really want to wear, that mountain you want to climb or that trip you want to take. Maybe the Camino de Santiago or something similar. Whatever you are working towards, make it visual and put it somewhere you will see it several times a day. You will be amazed by the impact it has on you and your motivation.

MEASURE

If you have followed me over the years, you will know that I have always believed in the power of measurement as a motivational tool. What gets measured gets changed; it is that simple. It really doesn't matter what you measure; just find something that is easy to measure and is relevant to you, track it and keep a note of it. It can be how many walks you do each week, for example. Or how many of Ireland's tallest peaks you have conquered. Or your resting heart rate. Whatever you like. I promise you that you will see a big difference in your motivation when you do it regularly. We'll have a look at some things that you can measure later on in the book (see page 80). When we measure things regularly, amazing results follow.

FRIEND OR PARTNER

Working together with someone is again something I have done for years and years. No matter what event I am trying to do or why, surrounding myself with people who do similar things and who are faster and fitter than I am has been so important to me succeeding. If you want to be healthier and make changes to your wellness, surrounding yourself with people healthier than you is a great way to do it. It is one of the many reasons that walking clubs are so popular and accessible. Having a group or a person to walk with can also give you an accountability partner. On days when you don't feel like it they help you, and you them – it is a win–win for all involved!

TECHNOLOGY

Technology and health is an area that is developing at a rapid rate, and it can be a great way to help you stay on track! Listening to a podcast or audio book when walking is a great way to pass the time; using Strava or MapMyWalk is a handy way to measure your distance and speed as well as a host of other things. If the budget allows, a GPS watch is great too. Meditation apps help you to be more mindful. But be careful: these are all really good ways to stay on track, but doom-scrolling while walking really isn't ideal, and being overly distracted when your mind is already racing isn't great either. We live in a world now where being bored or not distracted is rare and there is something incredibly powerful when we can just be, without anything to distract us, something that we will look at more later in the book.

TRAINING PLANS

In this section, I want to give you some simple training plans to help you step outside your comfort zone and reach for the stars. From a basic walking to 5k plan, a 10k plan and a full marathon walking plan, these training plans are tried and tested. Give yourself enough time to train, take it week by week and you will be amazed at how fast your fitness improves.

COUCH TO 5K

Here is a great couch to 5k programme to follow for those just starting out on their walking journey. This plan is for seven weeks, but you can shorten it by a week or two if you like.

COUCH TO 5K	WALK 1 EASY	WALK 2 FAST ON A NEW ROUTE	WALK 3 HILLY ROUTE
WEEK 1	20 mins	20 mins	30 mins
WEEK 2	20 mins	25 mins	35 mins
WEEK 3	25 mins	30 mins	40 mins
WEEK 4	30 mins	30 mins	50 mins
WEEK 5	30 mins	35 mins	60 mins
WEEK 6	35 mins	45 mins	70 mins
WEEK 7	30 mins	20 mins	5k

10K PLAN

So you've mastered the 5k walks and now you want to push yourself a little further. This training plan will take you to 10k over six weeks, so why not sign up for a 10k event to give yourself a great goal to work towards?

10K PLAN	WALK 1 FAST	WALK 2 HILLY ROUTE	WALK 3
WEEK 1	30 mins	45 mins	1 hour
WEEK 2	30 mins	45 mins	1 hour 15 mins
WEEK 3	45 mins	45 mins	1 hour 30 mins
WEEK 4	45 mins	45 mins	2 hours
WEEK 5	30 mins	45 mins	1 hour 30 mins
WEEK 6	30 mins	30 mins	**10k**

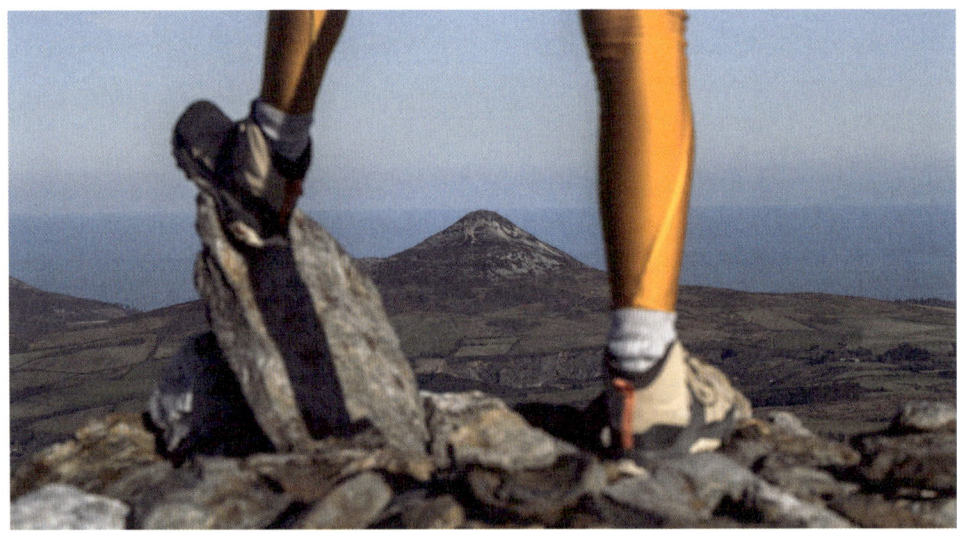

MARATHON PLAN

You would be amazed at just how many people walk marathons. It is a great way to see a city and a great goal to work towards. Yes, it is a little scary, but with some hard work you will get there. I have so many clients who have walked several marathons and it's something almost anyone can do!

Here's a really simple training plan.

MARATHON PLAN	WALK 1 FAST	WALK 2 HILLY ROUTE	WALK 3
WEEK 1	30 mins	45 mins	1 hour
WEEK 2	30 mins	45 mins	1 hour 30 mins
WEEK 3	30 mins	45 mins	1 hour 30 mins
WEEK 4	30 mins	45 mins	2 hours
WEEK 5	45 mins	45 mins	3 hours
WEEK 6	45 mins	1 hour	3 hours
WEEK 7	45 mins	1 hour	3 hours
WEEK 8	45 mins	1 hour	4 hours
WEEK 9	1 hour	1 hour	4 hours
WEEK 10	1 hour	1 hour	5 hours
WEEK 11	1 hour	1 hour	5 hours
WEEK 12	1 hour	1 hour	4 hours
WEEK 13	1 hour	1 hour	4 hours
WEEK 14	45 mins	45 mins	3 hours
WEEK 15	45 mins	45 mins	2 hours
WEEK 16	30 mins	30 mins	**Marathon**

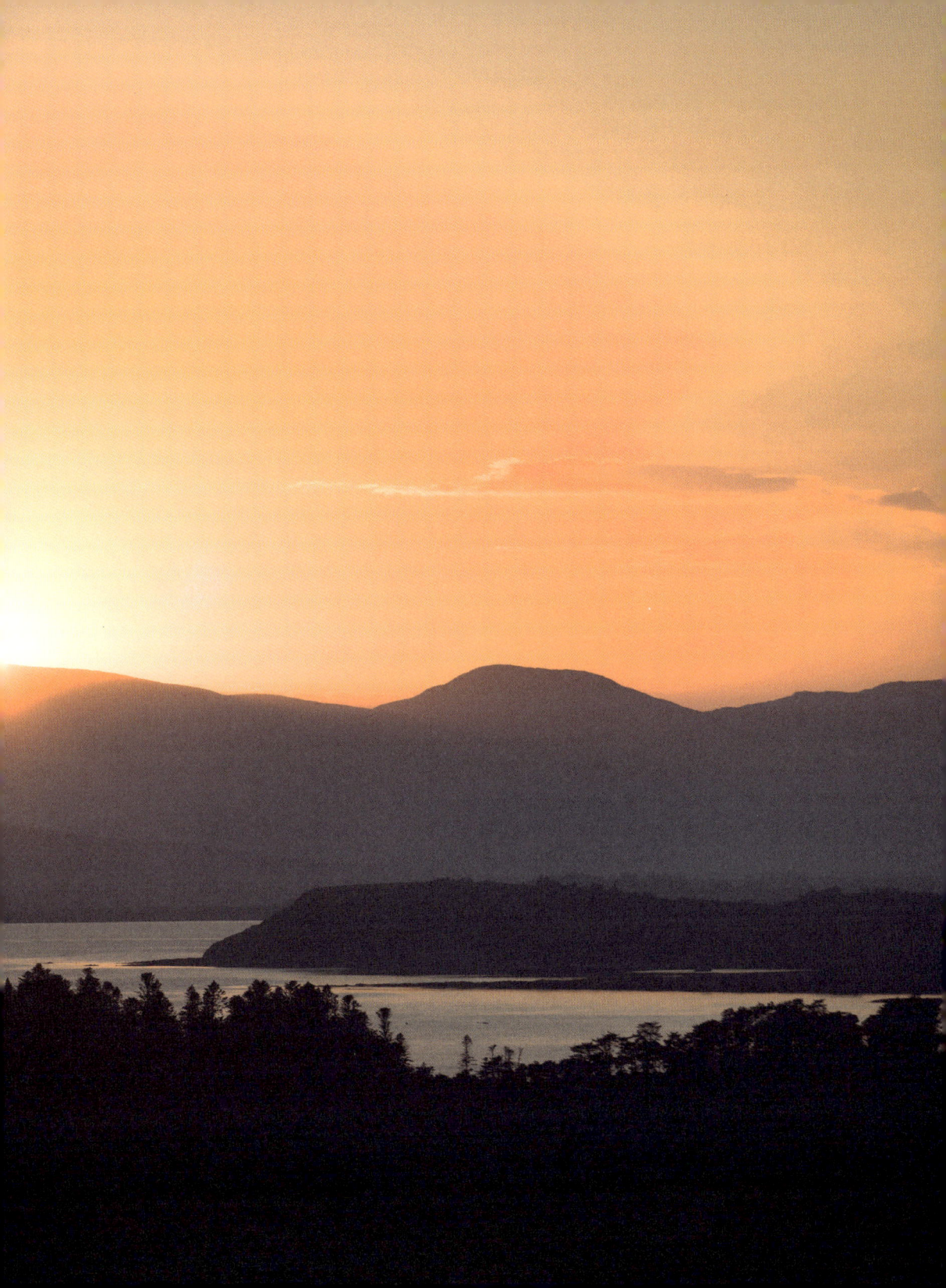

TIPS TO HELP YOU STAY ON TRACK

First of all, remember that Rome wasn't built in a day. Results take time. Anyone who tells you differently is not telling the truth. Pick a goal that you can work towards over time and as long as you are getting closer you are winning! You might like to complete some of the walks listed in the book, walk a marathon or do something you have always wanted to do.

+ When you fall off the wagon – and chances are this will happen at some stage – remember that no one's perfect and that change is hard. The key thing is to get back on track as soon as possible. You need to draw a line in the sand, accept the fact that you had a bad day or week and move forward. There is no point beating yourself up over it and feeling even worse. Just remember that everyone has bad days and moving on quickly is the best thing that you can do.

+ Don't just settle for average. When you are setting your goal, or setting a new one, having achieved the first, why not aim for something epic, something huge, something that you will be able to achieve even though it's a big leap? All too often we settle for the normal, the average, when we are in fact capable of so much more. As they say, reach for the stars!

+ Build a positive network. Those around you will directly impact how you feel, look and think. Surround yourself with people who will help to push your boundaries, your goals and your abilities. Surround yourself with the people you want to become, not those who can drag you down or restrict you from achieving your best.

+ Do it today! Do it now, write it down, text it to a friend, call someone and commit to the goal. Don't put it off or wait another week. Make that commitment now, today, that you are going to make the change, to register for that event, and you are going to do everything in your power to make it happen. Leave no stone unturned!

SIMPLE WAYS TO KEEP GETTING FITTER

These simple tips will stop that frustrating plateau; they will keep you working towards your goal and keep your body changing, giving you the results you want. Bodies are amazing – they adapt all the time to the environment they are placed in – so if you don't change anything about your walks or your workouts, it is no surprise that you begin to feel that you aren't making any progress. Try these simple tips to make the most of your walks!

KEEP UP THE INTENSITY

You should always feel that you are pushing your body in the sessions. As you get fitter, up the intensity, work harder and keep your heart rate up. You could use a heart rate monitor to check this. Ideally your heart should be working at a rate of 135–155 beats per minute. You should be getting out of breath but still able to hold a conversation. You could also try high-intensity interval training, which is fantastic, using two speeds or two effort levels and working between the two types of intensity. This can be great if you are short on time. Walking at an easy pace for, say, one minute and then as fast as you can for one minute will produce a really good workout, and as you get fitter and faster, keep pushing the pace. You can change up the time to suit your fitness level.

VARY YOUR WALKS

If you walk the same route at the same pace time and time again, your rate of adaptation will slow down, to the point at which you just won't be seeing any difference at all to your fitness, your body or your strength. Yes, that walk is providing some benefits, but not as many as you could get by varying it. In my opinion you should be changing your walks as often as possible, to keep your body adapting and getting results. You could change anything; the route, the pace, your walking partner, anything at all!

DON'T OVERTRAIN

If you do too much your body can begin to shut down; as a result, your progress will slow down. Overtraining is one of the key elements of the plateau effect, but how do you know if you're overtraining? You may be tired, grumpy, demotivated, sore after easy sessions, and your appetite may increase or decrease. These are some of the obvious symptoms. You can also use your resting heart rate as a guide, checking your pulse in the morning. If your resting pulse is consistently higher over a few days, you will know that you are overtraining. Pretty simple. If this happens, just ease back on the training, rest your body for a while, and when you feel like training again do just that!

HILLS

Hills are your best friend when it comes to getting great results. Add hills into your walks and watch what happens to your progress. It isn't just going up hills that helps: walking downhill is great for your core and your quads too.

WATCH YOUR PROTEIN LEVELS

If you find that you are taking a long time to recover from your walks, especially after upping your intensity, make sure you are getting enough protein in your diet to help you recover. Most people should aim for 1–1.5g of protein per kilogram body weight per day. That can go up to 2g per kilogram body weight if you are really active.

HOW TO WALK MORE WHEN YOU ARE BUSY

Let's face it: life has never been busier. Longer workdays, longer commutes and busy social lives mean that getting healthy and trying to fit exercise into your day has become harder and harder. It's something we see in every company we work with when we do corporate wellness work, and with our personal training clients too. Being too busy is actually a valid excuse when you are struggling to get healthy.

I know all too well that being too busy is a valid excuse. Sometimes I leave the house at 5 a.m. and often don't get back until eight or nine at night, after a busy day of personal training sessions with clients, meetings, writing and lectures. I have had to work out how to make sure that my own routine doesn't suffer when I am so busy. These are the ways I make it work.

For years I moved my sessions all the time to fit everything else in, more often than not missing those sessions. Now I spend time looking at my diary over the weekend and scheduling in my own training. I keep that time for myself and prioritise it, ensuring I get my training done at the times I have pencilled it in. If you respect your own time and fitness it will impact positively on everything around you. So sit down, plan those walks and commit to sticking to them.

Sometimes people don't exercise because it takes too long. So why not make your walks shorter, harder or maybe hillier? You will realise what you can do in just 30 minutes of your lunchbreak outside or on a treadmill. Those 30-minute sessions add up and make a big difference to your overall health.

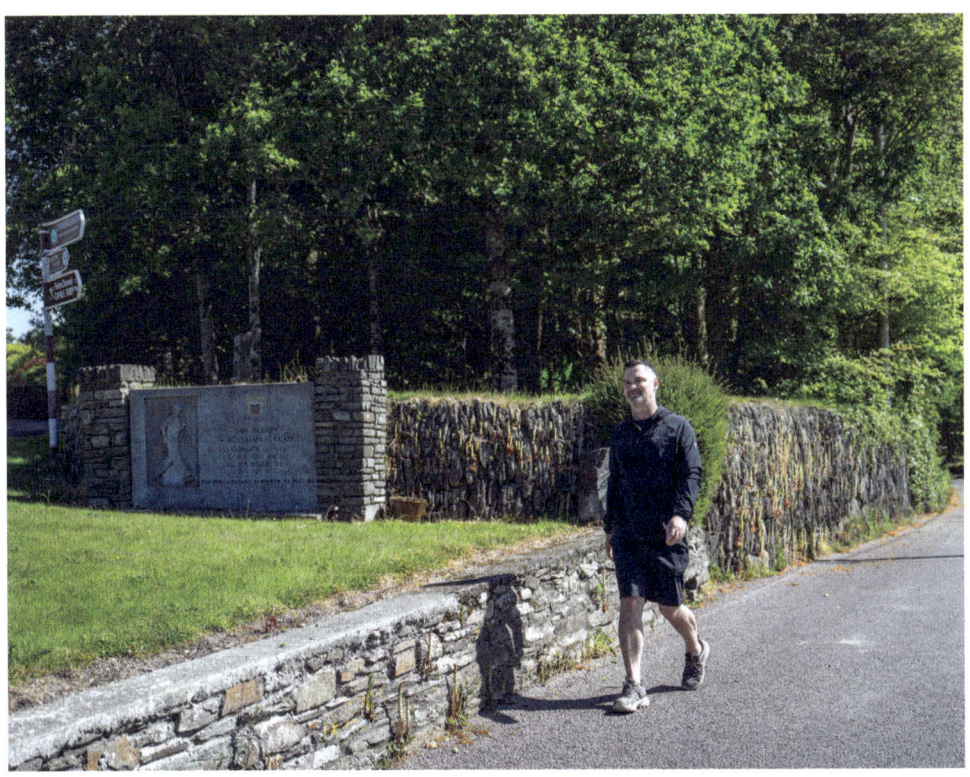

WHAT HAPPENS IF YOU GET INJURED?

When you are exercising, there is always a chance of picking up an injury, at any level of fitness. Depending how you deal with this injury, you can slow down or speed up your recovery. By applying the RICE principles (rest, ice, compression and elevation) you can ensure that you will be back training as soon as possible, and reduce the risk of doing further damage to yourself. It can be so hard to deal with injuries, but by using these principles you will be safe in the knowledge that you are doing your best.

+ *Rest*: Rest is vital to protect the injured muscle, tendon or ligament from further injury, as the more movement you place upon that area the worse your injury may become. Although this can be the most frustrating part, it is one of the most essential.
+ *Ice:* When icing an injury, choose a cold pack, crushed ice or a bag of frozen peas wrapped in a thin towel to provide cold to the injured area. This provides short-term pain relief and also limits swelling by reducing blood flow to the area. When icing injuries, never apply ice directly to the skin and never leave ice on an injury for more than 20 minutes at a time as you can damage your skin with ice burn. Every two minutes, take the ice pack off the skin and check for soreness or extreme redness – these can be signs of ice burn. Another great tip for reducing swelling is arnica cream or tablets.
+ *Compression:* Compression helps limit and reduce swelling around the injured area, which may delay healing. Some people also experience pain relief from compression. You can apply the compression yourself or pick up a support from your local chemist. If you experience throbbing, or if the wrap just feels too tight, it's important to remove the bandage and re-wrap the area so the bandage is a little looser. If it is too tight you will be reducing blood flow to the area, which will slow down the recovery process dramatically.
+ *Elevation:* Elevating an injury helps control swelling by improving circulation in the area. It's most effective when the injured area is raised above the level of the heart. So, if you injure an ankle, try lying on your bed with your foot propped on one or two pillows to get the leg elevated and the blood flowing back towards the body. If it's an arm injury, try to keep the arm up above chest level, even for short periods at a time, as this will reduce the initial swelling quite quickly.

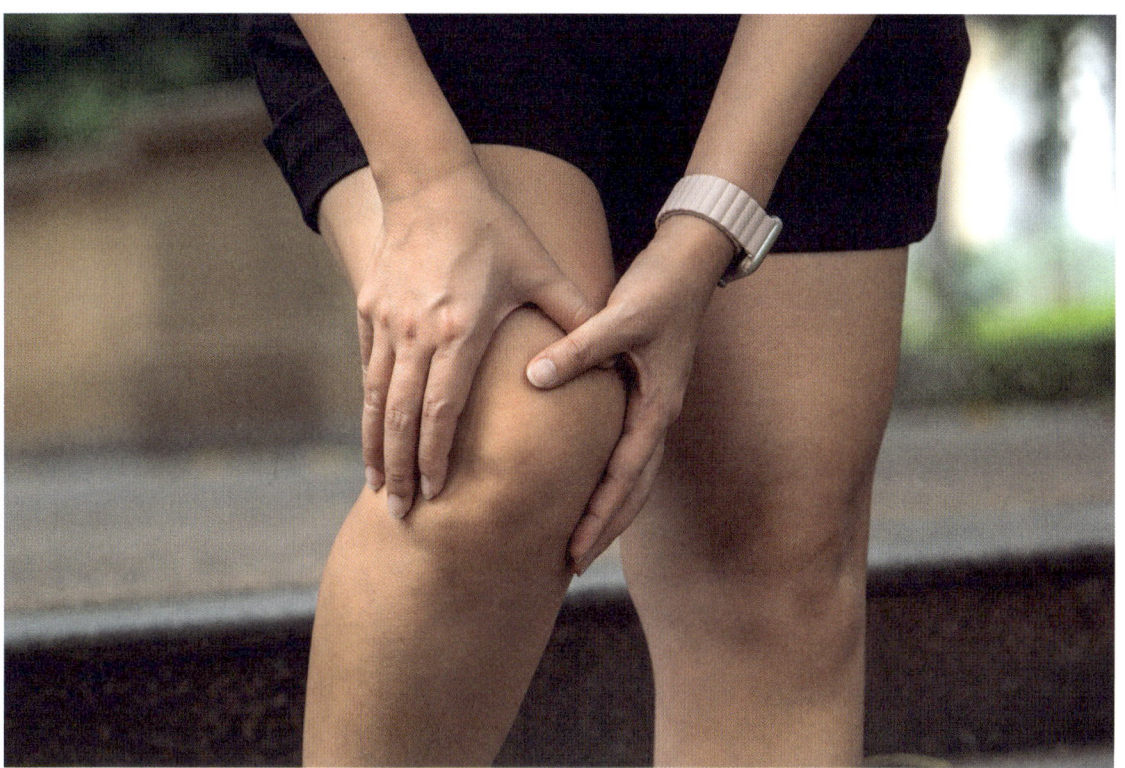

After a day or two of treatment, many sprains, strains and other injuries will begin to heal and get better. But if your pain or swelling does not decrease after 48 hours, make an appointment to see your GP or go straight to the hospital/Swiftcare clinic if you are really worried.

Once the healing process has begun, light massage may reduce the formation of scar tissue and improve tissue healing. You may also need to see a physiotherapist to aid the recovery process and give you exercises to do at home to increase the strength in the affected area.

You can begin gentle stretching after all swelling has subsided. Try to work the entire range of motion of the injured joint or muscle, but be extremely careful not to force a stretch, or you risk re-injury to the area. Keep in mind that a simple stretch should never cause pain. If it does, you know that you are pushing your body too far.

Remember, if you're not a physio yourself, the internet can be a very confusing source of information about stretches and healing. If you are even slightly in doubt, you should always consult a professional who knows what they are doing.

These simple tips will get you back walking and training quicker than ever, keeping you motivated and back exercising as soon as possible.

STRETCHING

Flexibility is really important for your overall health. Doing some simple stretches throughout the day can make a difference to your health, and it's good to do some stretches at the end of your walk too. Some people like to stretch at the start of a walk, but with most of my clients I get them to do a slightly slower pace to warm up the body at the start of the walk and then push the pace when they feel they have loosened up.

Here are some of the reasons you need to stretch:

+ Reduce stress
+ Reduce your medical bills
+ Improve your lean tissue
+ Lower the risk of cardiovascular disease
+ Lower the risk of injury
+ Improve mobility
+ Release endorphins
+ Lower the risk of lower-back pain
+ Keep you exercising when the weather is bad
+ Lower cholesterol
+ Reduce the risk of falls.

As reported by Howard LeWine in the *Harvard Medical Journal*:

> **Stretching keeps the muscles flexible and healthy, and we need that flexibility to maintain a range of motion in the joints. Without it, the muscles shorten and become tight. Then, when you call on the muscles for activity, they are unable to extend all the way. That puts you at risk for joint pain, strains, and muscle damage. Regular stretching keeps muscles long, lean, and flexible, and this means that exertion won't put too much force on the muscle itself. Healthy muscles also help a person with balance problems avoid falls.**

Here are some really simple stretches to try at home yourself.

YOGA UPPER BODY BENDS

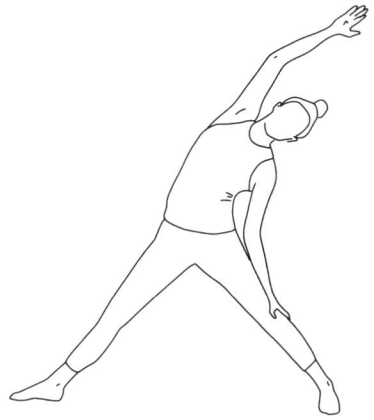

Start with your feet wider than shoulder width apart. Place one hand at the side of your leg and the other straight up in the air. Now stretch the arm in the air across towards your opposite shoulder and allow the hand on your leg to slide down the leg as you do so. Hold for 15 seconds and then change leg. Repeat for three sets.

SHOULDER ROLLS

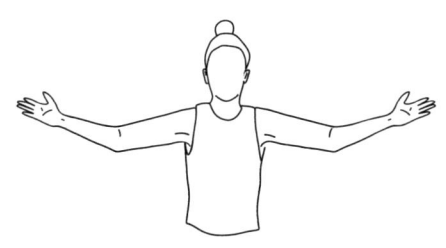

These are great to loosen up the shoulder joints and muscles.

Start with your feet together, and hands together. Keeping your arms straight, roll your arms back in big circles ten times and then roll forward for ten. These should be done slowly. Aim to stretch your arms out as far as possible. Repeat for three sets.

TRICEP STRETCH

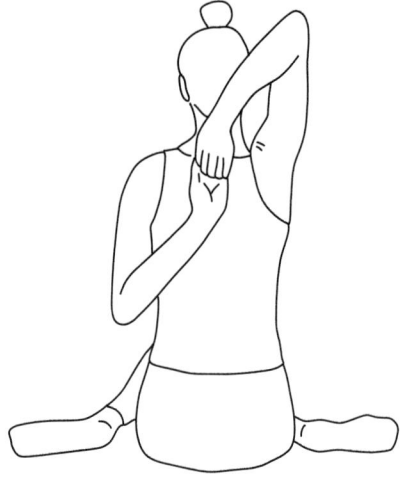

The triceps at the back of the arm can get quite tight and need a good stretch.

You can do this stretch either standing with your feet together or sitting on the ground, as in the illustration. Straighten your left arm above your head and your right arm by your side. Now bend your left arm behind your head and try to touch your hands in the centre of your back. If you can't touch your hands, don't worry, just get a towel between your hands and move your hands up the towel as you get more flexible. Hold the stretch for 15 seconds, then change hands.

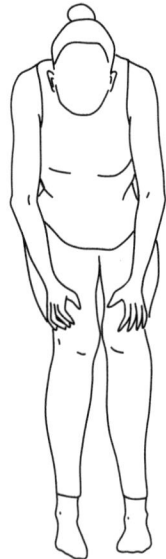

KNEE ROLLS

This is one of my favourite stretches and it's one of the simplest.

Place your feet together, knees together, and place your hands on the front of your knees. Now just roll your knees in a circular motion to the left for ten and then to the right for ten. These movements should be easy and gentle; the idea is to loosen out the ligaments, tendons and muscles around the knee joint.

HAMSTRING STRETCH

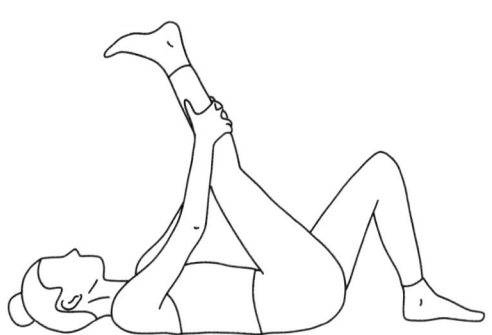

The hamstrings are a big muscle group at the back of the leg and if they become tight it can make you more prone to lower-back problems.

You start this stretch by lying on the ground. With one knee bent, straighten the opposite leg in the air and place your hands behind your leg to create the stretch. Hold for 15 seconds and then change leg. Repeat for three sets.

QUAD STRETCH

The quad is at the front of the leg and is a seriously big muscle group. This is one of the simplest ways to stretch it out.

Lie on your left side, take your right ankle in your right hand and bring your right heel up to your bum. Hold for 15 seconds and then roll over onto the opposite leg and do the same. Repeat for three sets.

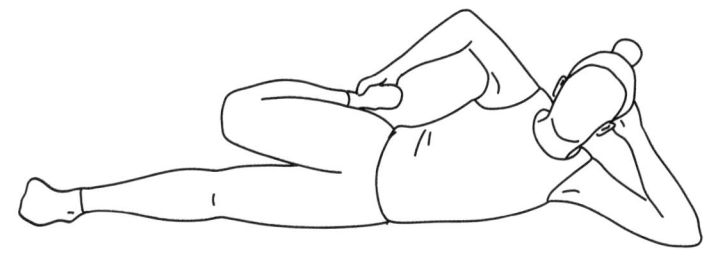

This stretching routine is easy to do and will gently loosen out all parts of your body. Remember, it's important not to push the body to the point of pain; just ease into it, relax and stretch the body a little, and you will be surprised at how quickly you loosen up.

Do these stretches any time during the day, or habit-stack them with something that you always do every day, such as brushing your teeth.

SORENESS AND HOW TO REDUCE IT

Muscles are made up of fibres, and when you do something different you place these fibres under pressure, forcing them to tear minutely. Over time, they then grow back together stronger and firmer. This process is what causes that muscle soreness that you sometimes feel after a walk. Here are some really simple ways to reduce the soreness.

STRETCHING

Doing some simple stretches after your walk doesn't have to take very long, or be really hard. In the previous section we looked at some really good stretches. They will help you to recover faster and prevent DOMS (delayed onset muscle soreness).

Here are some more simple stretches you can try specifically at the end of your walk, especially after a hard, fast or hilly walk, when you will really feel the impact of the session. So try some of these stretches and hold them for 20–30 seconds. You can do them as many times as you like.

STANDING QUAD STRETCH

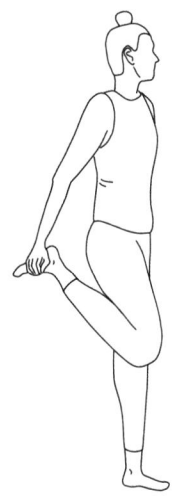

This stretch is great for your hip flexors and your quadriceps muscles at the front of your leg. They are big muscle groups and do a lot of the work when you walk, especially up and down hills. For this stretch, you can hold on to something for stability just in case you fall while doing it.

Standing tall and straight, with your legs shoulder-width apart, bend one leg at the knee and use your hand to reach back and hold your foot behind you, against your bum, or as close to it as you can get without straining yourself too much. Then repeat with the other leg. This is a stretch that you will get better at over time.

CALF STRETCH

Your calves, at the backs of the lower parts of your legs, between your ankles and your knees, play a big part in walking, so it's very important to keep them happy.

Start on the floor with your arms straight, your hands on the floor and your knees bent. Extend one leg straight back and place the ball of your foot on the floor. Press your heel away from you to start the stretch. Hold for 15 seconds, then change leg.

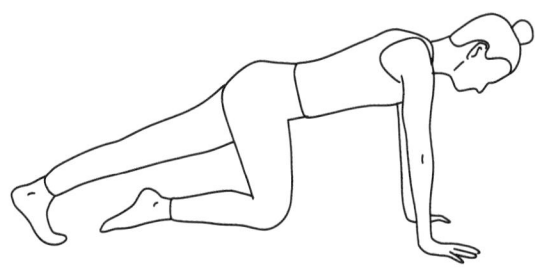

HAMSTRING STRETCH

Hamstrings are notorious for tightening up and can often cramp up, so it's important to stretch these after a workout. Hamstrings and back pain are also linked – if you have tight hamstrings there is a good chance you will have some lower-back pain too.

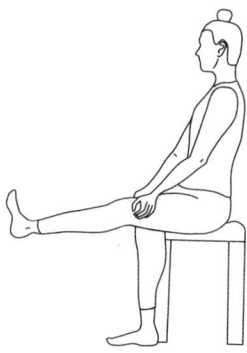

For this stretch, sit on a chair with your feet slightly apart and flat on the floor in front of you. Raise one leg, keeping your leg straight. While holding onto the chair for balance with the opposite hand, reach forward towards your foot with the other hand. If possible, hold onto your foot and feel the stretch through the back of your leg, and hold for around 30 seconds before repeating with the other leg. You can also use a towel to help you do this if you can't keep your leg straight: loop the towel around the back of the foot and hold the ends in your hand.

HIP STRETCH

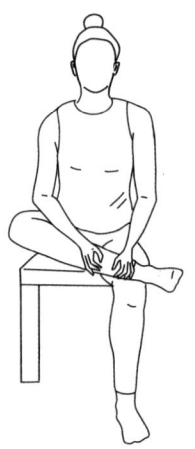

Stretching out your hips improves mobility and flexibility. They can be surprisingly tight and that can really impact not just your walking but your life. This stretch works on the muscle group located near the top of your thigh, the hip flexors.

Sit on a chair, raise your right leg and place your right ankle on top of your left knee. Using the chair for balance, gently lean forward to feel the stretch in the back of your thigh and buttock. Hold this position for 30 seconds, then repeat with the other leg. Don't push the muscles too far; ease into it, and it will get easier over time as you become more flexible.

POSTERIOR SHOULDER STRETCH

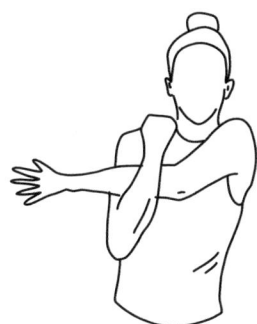

This shoulder stretch works on your shoulder muscles and upper-back muscles. You will be surprised just how much work your shoulders and back do when you're walking, so try this simple stretch.

Standing tall with your feet shoulder-width apart, bring one arm across your body and use the other arm to gently hold and push it in towards your body. Hold this position for 30 seconds before swapping arms.

Stretching doesn't have to be hard or take ages, and adding these stretches to your routine will make a big difference to your walk and to how you feel. By keeping your muscles supple and flexible, not only are you helping to reduce your chances of muscle aches, you're also reducing the risk of injury.

If you find stretching boring or struggle to do it, you might find it useful to join a local yoga class. It is something I do myself: I find going to a class and having someone tell me what to do means I get a really good session done, even when I don't want to do it.

WHY WALKING IS THE PERFECT EXERCISE IF ...

YOU'RE WORRIED THAT YOU'RE TOO OLD

You are never too old to start exercising, and including strength-based training is the best way you can improve your health at any age. Just start slow and build it up.

YOU FEEL UNFIT

No matter how unfit you are, fear not. You are never too unfit to start. You just need to make small changes to your health, small changes that will get easier over time and will enable you to progress to harder workouts that deliver even more benefits. Any exercise will improve your fitness and your health, and you will be amazed at how the body can change over time and improve, so just start small, build it up as you feel you can and watch what happens.

YOU FIND THE IDEA OF INTENSIVE EXERCISE DAUNTING

Often intensive exercise programmes can be too hard, leaving you sore and demotivated. Jumping into a routine when you haven't exercised for a long time always puts you at risk, so aim to follow a plan that helps you get fitter the right way each week. If you find it too difficult, reduce the repetitions of the exercise or the sets and increase the amount of breaks you take.

YOU'RE NOT SURE WHERE TO START

This can actually be the scariest part of exercise for many people – where to start and what to do. Let me help you. The reality is that starting with something you enjoy is good. Then you're more likely to progress as you get fitter.

YOU'RE WORRIED ABOUT GETTING INJURED

For anyone – of any fitness level or age – there is always a risk of injury. But you reduce this risk by following the right plan, stretching at the end of each session, taking a break when you need it, resting when required and also seeking a GP's check-up before you start exercising.

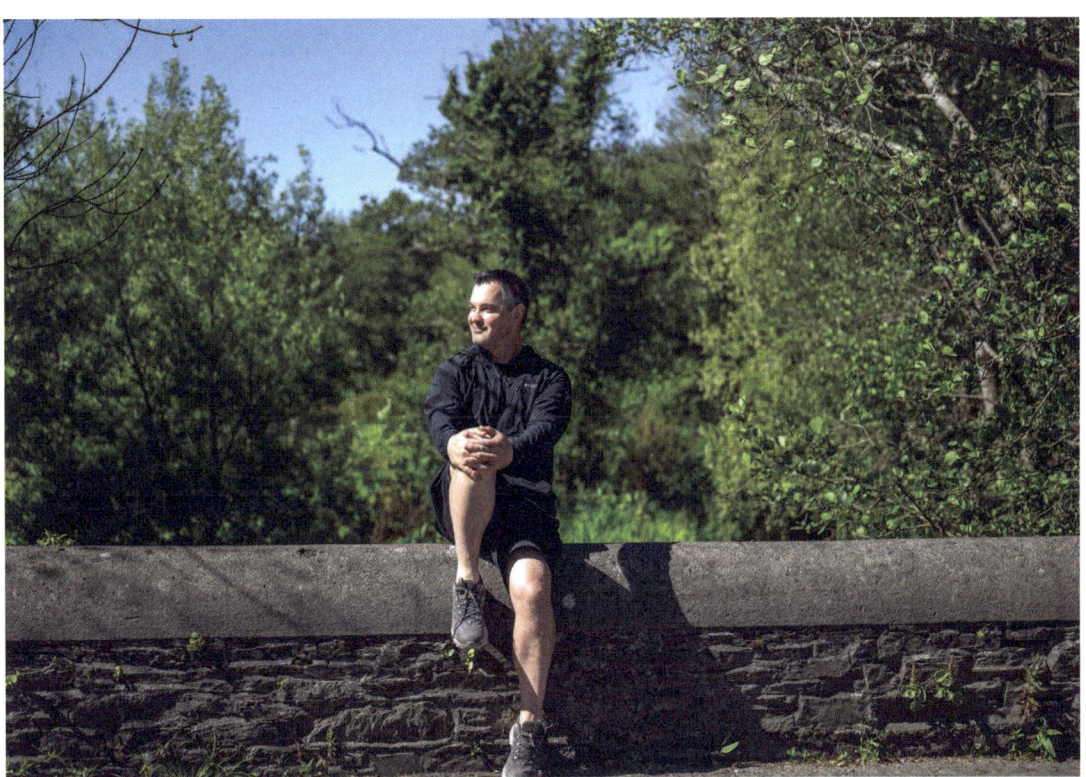

By now I hope I have shown you that walking is a powerful, simple and effective way of making a real difference, not only to you but also to those around you. It is something that everyone can do and every single step makes a big difference. No matter what age you are or how unfit you are, the walking effect is something truly special.

ANXIETY, STRESS AND WALKING

We know that people with anxiety and high stress levels tend to move less, which in turn increases their levels of anxiety and stress. Any movement, no matter how big or small, will dramatically impact anxiety and stress levels. Every step you take will produce endorphins, helping to reduce anxiety and fatigue and boosting your mood.

'There is emerging evidence that walking ... lowers the risk of depression and the development and progression of Alzheimer's disease and other related dementias,' says Roger Fielding PhD, leader of the nutrition, exercise physiology and sarcopenia team at the Jean Mayer USDA Human Nutrition Research Center on Aging at Tufts University.

A study of over 78,000 people found that walking 3,800 steps per day reduced the risk of dementia by 25 per cent. Walking 9,826 steps per day (about five miles) reduced the risk of dementia by 50 per cent.

The research amazes me – how walking can create change within the body and the mind, even when it comes to such serious illnesses.

A paper by John Ratey MD, an associate clinical professor of psychiatry at Harvard Medical School and an internationally recognised expert in neuropsychiatry, reported that:

+ Engaging in exercise diverts you from the very thing you are anxious about.
+ Moving your body decreases muscle tension, lowering the body's contribution to feeling anxious.
+ Getting your heart rate up changes brain chemistry, increasing the availability of important anti-anxiety neurochemicals, including serotonin, gamma aminobutyric acid (GABA), BDNF and endocannabinoids.
+ Exercise activates frontal regions of the brain responsible for executive function, which helps control the amygdala, the part of the brain that reacts or imagined threats to our survival.
+ Exercising regularly builds up resources that bolster resilience against stormy emotions.

The best part of these findings is that the exercise you do doesn't have to be incredibly strenuous or hard. Any level of intensity will deliver these mood-related benefits.

WALKING AND STRENGTH

Losing strength is one of the fastest-growing problems in our society. We lose strength as we get older. The more we sit and the less we move, the more muscle and strength we lose. Being sedentary accelerates the ageing process, puts people at more risk of trips and falls and makes even the most basic of daily functions hard. Walking is one of nature's ways of keeping us strong.

With every step you take, you are asking your body to stay strong, to adapt, to keep you safe and healthy. Every muscle in your body has to work to stay strong with every step that you take. As we get older it is 'use it or lose it' time.

Walking, by nature, is what keeps us well, keeps us young and keeps us strong. The cycle of ageing accelerates when the moving decreases. When you start parking as close as possible to where you're going, doing less housework, asking someone else to bring in the logs in winter, avoiding the gardening – these are the simple life choices that will accelerate the ageing process. The less you do, the faster you age. Carry in the logs. Keep going with the housework. Do as much as you can for as long as you can. That's the secret to staying strong, living not just longer but better, and maintaining your independence. It is a choice. An opportunity to live better. Stop choosing the easy option of moving less and control your own ageing by choosing to keep going, even if some jobs take you longer as you get older. Walking is the key to this.

WHY BE STRONG?

Put very simply, strength is life. Strength is one of the ultimate factors in living better and living longer; and walking more is one of the best ways to stay strong. In a study by Kalyani et al., the researchers found that both low muscle mass and poor muscle strength are important risk factors for disability and potentially mortality in individuals as they get older. Many chronic diseases could also accelerate the loss of muscle mass and strength. This is why it is so important to stay strong and maintain your muscle as you age!

WHAT HAS WALKING GOT TO DO WITH STRENGTH?

Walking has everything to do with strength. It is the easiest way to keep yourself strong. Even just standing will do that. It is sitting that is bad for our health.

Let's have a look at it in a little more detail. Walking is an aerobic exercise: it gets your heart pumping. When you walk fast you get out of breath and because of that, many people think of the health benefits of walking as being cardiovascular alone.

But the reality is that the other benefits include arthritis relief, improved sleep, reduced stress, a boosted immune system, improved glucose control, stronger bones and greater levels of muscle mass in the body.

Walking will help you to build some muscle too. Muscles grow after being stressed enough to break down in the first place. This is why I am always asking people to challenge their bodies somewhat when they are moving. Challenging the body requires it to repair the microtears in muscle by strengthening and reinforcing the areas around them.

While walking won't break down muscles the same way weight training does, it can break down muscles in some muscle groups, causing them to tone and grow over time. This is especially true for people who may not exercise on a regular basis or are just getting started on their fitness journey. Beyond strengthening muscles, walking can also help maintain the muscle mass you already have.

'Muscle loss, called sarcopenia, happens with age,' explains Michael Fredericson MD, director of the Physical Medicine and Rehabilitation division of Stanford University. 'But regular exercise, including walking, can help reduce its effects.'

WHICH MUSCLE GROUPS DOES WALKING BUILD?

Walking works your core, your quads (the fronts of the legs), your hamstrings (the backs of the legs), your glutes (your bum) and your calves. It also helps to strengthen the ligaments and tendons of the lower body. Walking correctly can help to strengthen the postural muscles of the upper body as well. The degree to which these muscles grow will depend on several factors including gender, age, body mass, existing muscle strength, and whether you are walking on the flat or on an incline. If you really want to use walking as a way to get stronger, you have to add inclines – walking uphill and downhill – into your walk. One of the geographical features of Blue Zones – regions of the world where people have longer life expectancies – is that they are hilly. Yes, hills can make walking tough, but remember what they are doing for your strength.

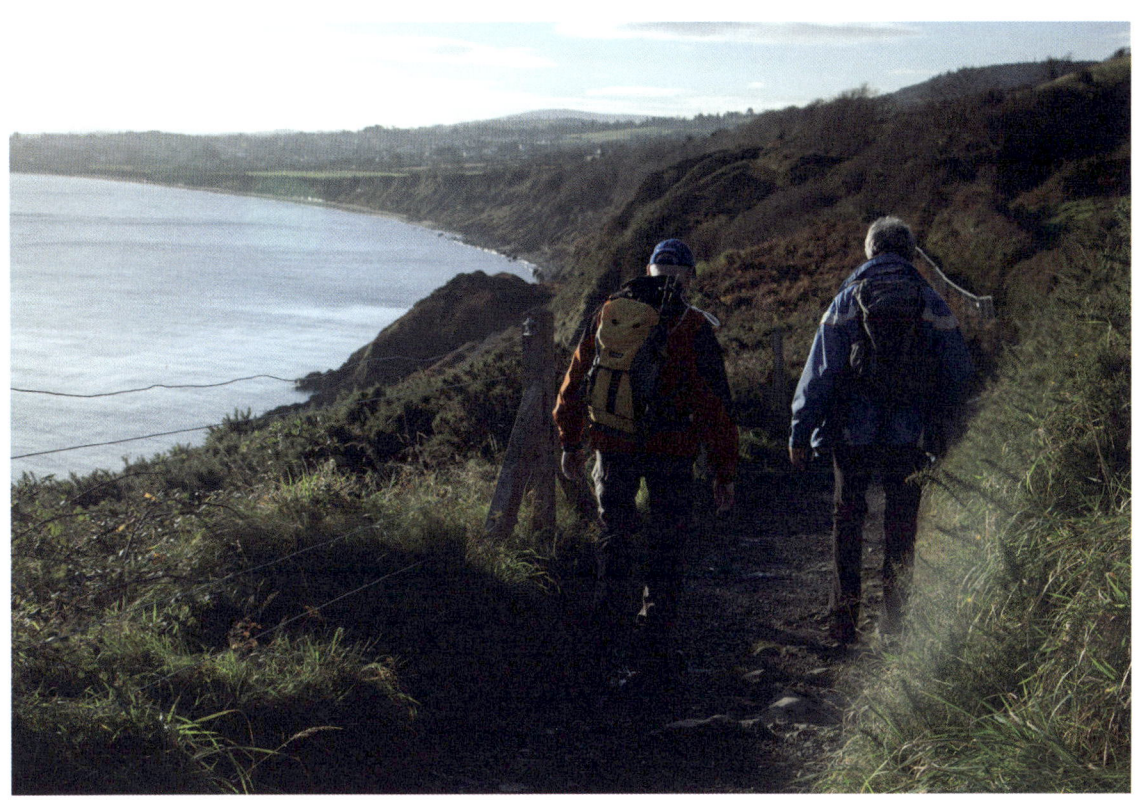

THE IMPORTANCE OF STAYING STRONG AS WE GET OLDER

Our chronological age and our bodies' age are two very different things. You may be 60 and fit, or 60 and unfit. Weight, muscle mass, fat mass, strength and bone strength are all ways of predicting your actual age. I have yet to meet one person who doesn't want to age better and healthier, yet so many people still don't do enough. One of the motivators I had for writing this book was to show you that walking is one of the key tools that we can all use every day to age better and age healthier.

A study by Zoltan Ungvari, a researcher into ageing health, found that the evidence overwhelmingly supports walking as a powerful anti-ageing intervention that can reduce the risk of chronic age-related diseases such as cardiovascular disease, hypertension, type 2 diabetes and cancer. Walking also improves pain and function in people with musculoskeletal disorders, promotes sleep and mental health and increases resilience. The study found that overall, walking is a simple and effective intervention that can be easily integrated into daily routines to promote healthy ageing and prevent chronic age-related diseases.

SIMPLE STRENGTH TESTS

I want to show you some really simple exercises that can help you stay strong and walk better. Walking is the body's weight-bearing movement, but if you add in some simple resistance training you will really see the difference. These exercises can make you even stronger, yet so few people do them. I'll take you through those exercises later, but first I want to begin with some really simple ways to measure your strength. What gets measured gets changed, so take a look at these strength tests below and don't just read them – try them yourself and see how you get on with them.

Measuring your strength levels is a direct way to measure your biological age and predict how you are going to age. These tests were developed by the sports science team in Dublin City University and we have used them for several years to track people's progress as they begin to get healthier and stronger. The changes we see in four weeks are incredible. Not only will you feel stronger but these tests will back up the feeling with visible evidence.

My advice is to take the tests, record your results and then take them again four weeks later. Hopefully you will see improvements in your results, but even just maintaining your numbers is good. These tests work for everyone, irrespective of age or fitness level.

With all of these tests, try to do as many as you can or hold them for long as you can. They are maximal tests. There are recommended numbers you should be able to achieve at different fitness levels, but in my opinion these can demotivate people, so I tend not to use them. If I can simply encourage you to take the test, I am proud and happy! Just see what you can do and aim to improve when you retest. I guarantee that it will keep you strong and when you see the numbers improve you will be more motivated too.

Let's take a look at how to do the different tests.

TIMED BALANCE TEST

What you need: A stopwatch and a level floor.

How to do the test: Flex your standing leg and really plant your foot into the ground. Feel the ground with your toes and spread them as best you can. Now cross your arms, raise your other leg and hold the position for 30 seconds with your eyes open (do this to ensure that you can safely perform the rest of the test). Repeat the same task for as long as possible with your eyes closed. Your time is up when you lose balance / if your standing foot moves / if you open your eyes / your non-standing foot touches the floor.

Take three attempts and record your best score.

UPPER-BODY STRENGTH TEST

What you need: Nothing but your body and a safe space that isn't too warm.

If you are male, you are required to do full press-ups to pass the test. But don't worry, if you can't do the test with a full press-up just stick with the modified until you feel up to the challenge of the full press-up.

If you are female, you can do modified press-ups.

Do as many press-ups as possible until exhaustion and be careful not to let your technique go. Count the total number of press-ups performed.

• Regular press-up technique

How to do the test: The starting position is face down with your weight distributed between your hands and feet, arms straight. Your body should be rigid and straight, and your hands are placed approximately shoulder-width apart. Lower your body until your chest nears the floor at the bottom of the movement, upper arms parallel with the ground, then return to the starting position.

- **Modified press-up technique**

How to do the test: Kneel on the floor. Put your hands on the floor, either side of your chest, and keep your back straight. Lower your chest down towards the floor, to the same level each time, either until your elbows are at right angles or your chest touches the ground.

LOWER-BODY STRENGTH TEST

What you need: A chair with a straight back and without armrests (e.g. a kitchen chair). Make sure the chair's on a level, flat surface. You could set it with its back against a wall so that the chair is safe and doesn't move.

How to do the test: Sit in the middle of the chair. Place your hands on the opposite shoulders, crossed at the wrists. Keeping your feet flat on the floor, your back straight and your arms against your chest, rise to a full standing position and then sit down again.

Repeat this for 30 seconds. Keep breathing all the way through. Be careful not to rush the test or bounce up and down: stay controlled and steady throughout. Count and record the number you complete.

CARDIOVASCULAR FITNESS TEST

What you need: A stopwatch (or a stopwatch app on your smartphone) and a fitness tracker or smart watch (e.g. a Fitbit or an app that records distance in kilometres or miles). Or, if you're using a pitch, you could have someone counting the amount of laps you do. Another option is to use your local running track, which will probably be 400 metres. Or you could take this test on a treadmill.

How to do the test: Time yourself as you walk or run for 12 minutes. Try to cover as much distance as you can. Measure the distance you've travelled over the 12 minutes using a fitness tracker or app.

Here's a table for you to record your results:

TEST	TIMED BALANCE TEST	UPPER-BODY STRENGTH TEST	LOWER-BODY STRENGTH TEST	CARDIOVASCULAR FITNESS TEST
TODAY Date: _____				
AFTER 1 MONTH Date: _____				
AFTER 2 MONTHS Date: _____				
AFTER 3 MONTHS Date: _____				
AFTER 4 MONTHS Date: _____				
AFTER 5 MONTHS Date: _____				
AFTER 6 MONTHS Date: _____				

WALKING AND WEIGHT LOSS

I have no doubt that some people will have bought this book because they want to improve their health and, as part of that, to lose weight. Weight has become something of a taboo subject in recent years, yet it is something that is so important for your health and wellness.

Knowing not just your weight but your body composition is really important. Both are key factors in healthy ageing. Being a healthy weight reduces bone and joint issues, reduces health-related risks, and lots more. Yet for some reason society is afraid to talk about it. So let's look at the reality. We are all a weight, and it is just a number. As we get older that number tends to change; it increases by, on average, a stone (roughly 6.3kg) per decade. When you carry more weight, you're putting more pressure on your joints.

Depending on your genetics you carry weight in different areas, and this is really important too. Weight carried around your middle is more dangerous than weight carried around your hips as it increases your risk of cardiovascular disease and other health-related issues. This visceral fat isn't the fat you can pinch, it's the fat that surrounds the internal organs inside the body. We can link it to pretty much every medical condition that there is. If you look around you at people of any age, especially the over-50s, look at where they carry their weight. The classic apple shape is all too common in Ireland, and a sign that the person is at a higher risk of cardiovascular disease and many other medical issues.

As well as knowing your weight, you should know your waistline measurement. Measure your waistline, around your bellybutton. If it's over 40 inches (101cm), aim to reduce it, ideally into the mid-thirties. Even if you can get it below 40 inches you will be doing really well and going a long way to improving your health.

Now, weight on its own is not the best health indicator because that number is made up of muscle and fat mass. These are two numbers that everyone should know. From our mid-thirties, as we gain weight, we start to gain more fat mass and lose muscle mass. You will know from reading the book this far that muscle mass is really important in ageing. If you know how much muscle you have and how much fat you have, you can track these numbers. If you are aiming to lose weight, you want to maintain muscle and lose body fat mass. To obtain these numbers, you need smart scales. Most will sync with an app on your phone and give you all the stats you need.

We lose weight by creating a calorie deficit. You simply expend more calories than you take in and, as a result, you lose weight. You create the deficit by eating better and moving more. That may seem over-simplified, and in some regards it is. Weight loss is challenging, but walking is a great tool in helping you to lose weight and change your body composition. There are exceptions to that rule – menopause, for example, changes all the rules – but the good news is that you can change your body composition at any age. Once you have your stats, it is time to work hard, walk hard and watch what happens.

It has also been shown that walking can even help to counteract the effects of obesity-promoting genes, something we are learning more about every year. A study of over 12,000 people by Harvard researchers showed that the effects of these genes were halved in participants who walked briskly for about an hour a day. So up the intensity of your walk and reap the rewards.

A pair of studies from the University of Exeter found that a 15-minute walk can curb cravings for chocolate and even reduce the amount of chocolate you eat in stressful situations. And the latest research confirms that walking can reduce cravings for and intake of a variety of sugary snacks. So walking can reduce cravings as well as being great exercise!

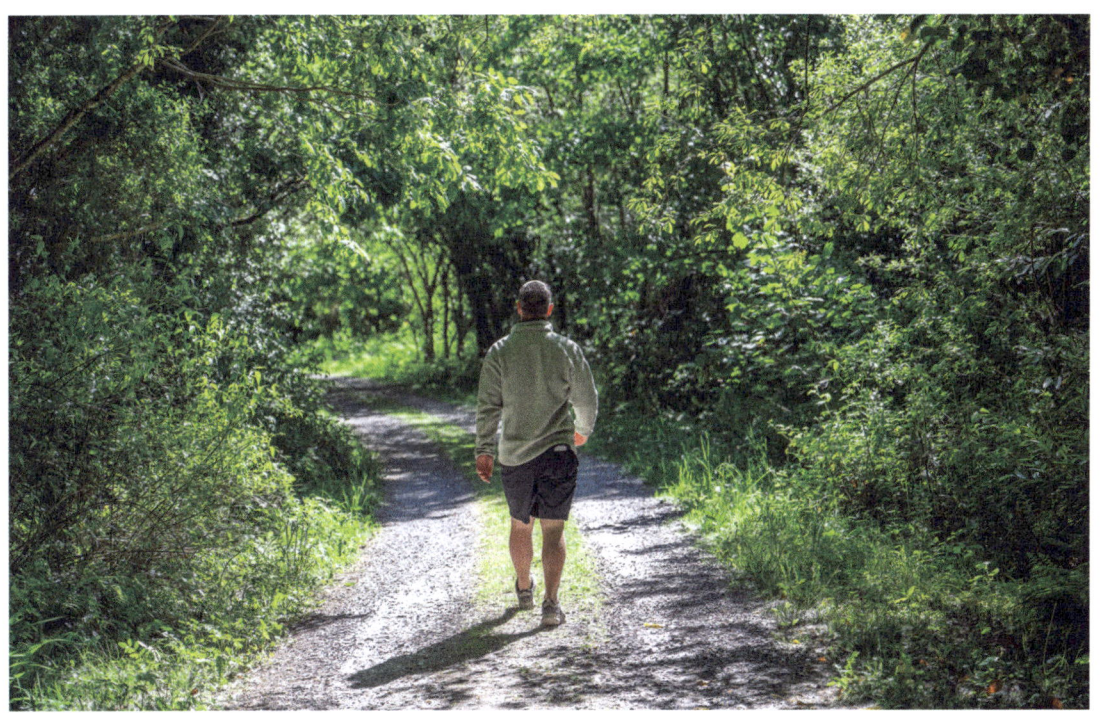

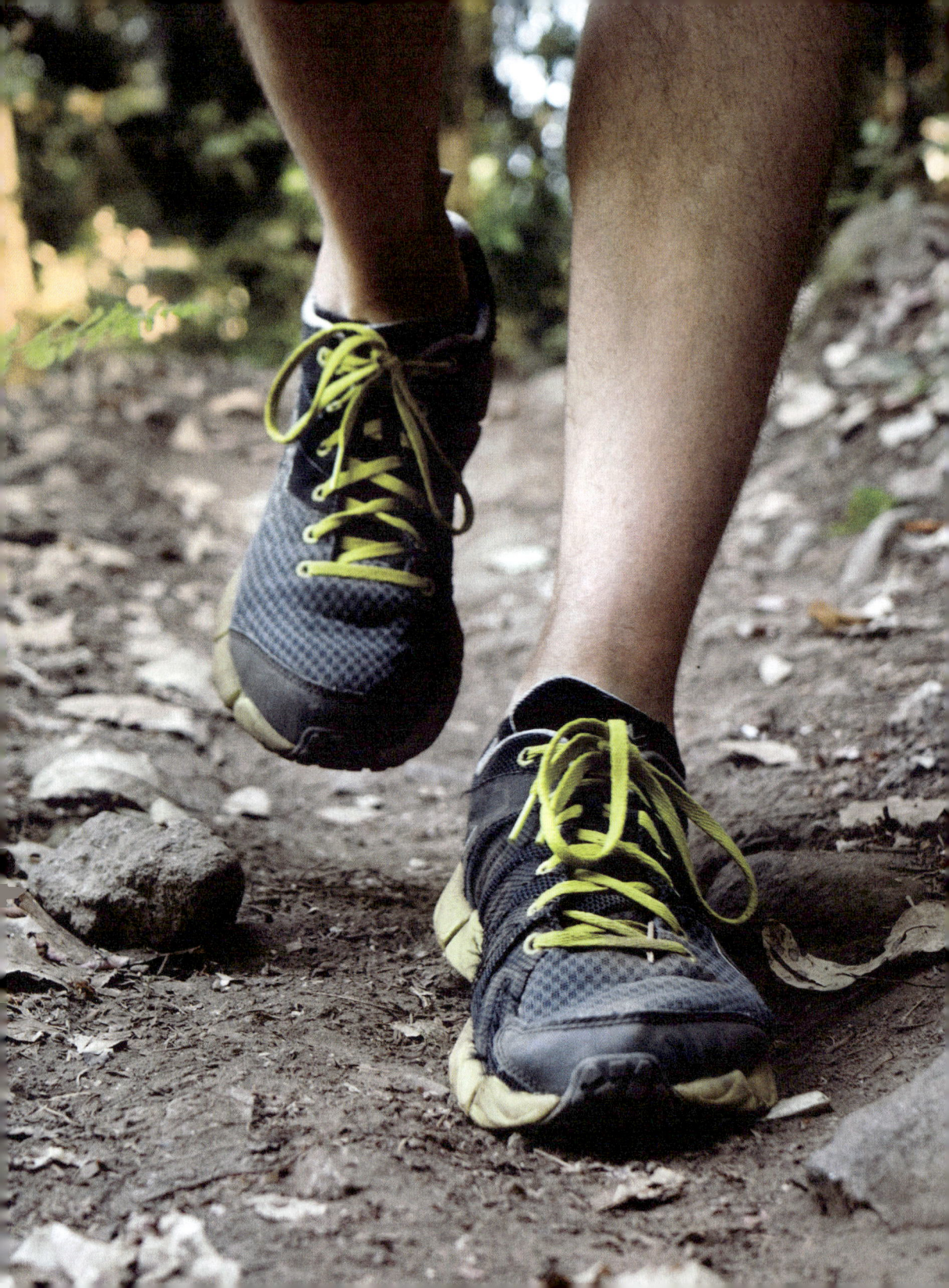

CHAPTER THREE

WHAT TO WEAR AND WHAT TO BRING

You don't need much to get a good walk in, but in this section I want to suggest what you might like to invest in to make the experience as enjoyable as possible. For some, walking in your day-to-day shoes will suffice, and that's cool, but I really believe that if you set yourself up as best you can you will get so much more out of it and you can really use walking to transform everything about your health. Don't worry – nothing I am recommending has to be expensive or complicated. So let's take a look at what you can add to your walk to make it even better.

WHY GEAR IS SO IMPORTANT

Picture the scene. Two people go out for a walk in the pouring rain. After a brisk 60-minute walk, they come back in very different states. One person is soaked to the bone, with heavy rain-drenched clothes, soggy feet and lots of chafing from clothing. The second person comes back dry, comfortable and feeling really good.

The difference between the two walkers is clothing and gear. If you really want walking to work for you, invest in the gear that will help you to walk no matter what the weather, because bad weather is something I can guarantee you we are always going to have.

SOCKS

Let's start with the feet. The socks you wear are going to make or break the comfort of your walk. Normal socks are generally made of some combination of cotton, nylon, polyester and wool, and these socks don't deal with sweat well; they get soggy, heavy and uncomfortable. They increase your chance of getting blisters. They are just not nice. Instead try sports socks, which will feel lighter and have a different texture. They are usually made of a blend of exclusively synthetic materials like nylon, polyester and spandex, which gives them more durability and flexibility and helps to deal with the sweat that comes from your feet when you move.

Hillwalking or hiking socks tend to be made out of merino wool or other sheep wool and synthetic fabric and they tend to be longer, heavier and with far more padding. They're designed to tackle harsher conditions, so they're great for that, but for a normal walk in the city or on roads, sports socks will do perfectly.

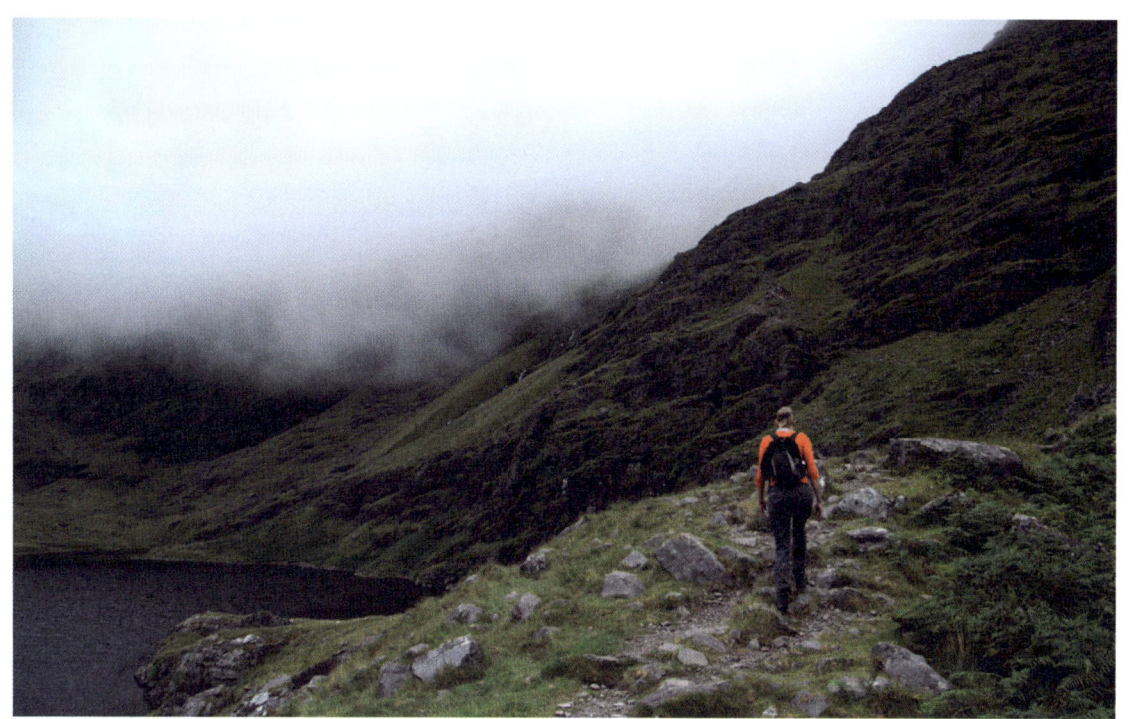

FOOTWEAR

You have four main choices here.

HIKING BOOTS

These are great for hiking in mountains or on muddy trails and beaches. They are comfortable, sturdy and offer really good support to the ankle. They are also generally waterproof, helping to keep your feet dry in bad weather. Don't buy your hiking boots online and don't pick a pair because you like the colour. You really need to get into a shop and get fitted for them properly, ideally when you're wearing hiking socks. Of the three choices, these are the most technical and expensive option so it is worth spending the time on getting the right pair. Once you do, they will last years.

TRAIL SHOES

Trail shoes are the hybrid of the footwear selection. Lighter than hiking boots and with way more support and grip than regular runners, they are a great all-round shoe for mixed trails and roads, and they also have better waterproof technology than runners. Again, it is worth getting these in person and having a proper fit done to make sure you get the right pair, especially if you plan on doing longer distances – your feet will swell when you up the distance.

RUNNERS

Then we have runners, the most popular choice. Most people pick their runners based on the brand or colour, but this is an area where you need to invest some time. When choosing runners you need to know your gait. Most sports stores offer a gait analysis service free of charge, and once you know what your foot type is you can make a much better decision when buying, whether online or from a shop.

Most people walk in one of three ways:

+ Supination – walking more on the outside of your foot
+ Pronation – walking more on the inside of your foot
+ Neutral – walking evenly across the foot when your foot hits the ground.

Different runners have different types of cushioning to support your foot, and it is important to know how your foot hits the ground so that you can choose the right runner to help you avoid injury in the long run.

BAREFOOT SHOES

Barefoot shoes have become incredibly popular in the last few years and I have two pairs myself. Essentially they are like a second skin, with a thin rubber sole and no arch support. The idea is that they give you a more natural walking experience. I find them comfortable and good to use for walking around the house or gardening, but I would not recommend them for long distances. If you are going to try them, then remember to slowly adjust to wearing them as they can cause a lot of leg and sometimes back pain if you do too much too soon.

CLOTHING

I am always fascinated when I see people walking in clothes that just make the whole experience far from enjoyable. Making better choices means that you will enjoy the walk so much more. It is a pretty simple switch, really, from clothes that hold on to sweat and rain to clothes that deal better with it. Heavy cotton tracksuits, T-shirts and jumpers get uncomfortable when they're wet and, like badly chosen socks, increase the risk of chafing, which will eventually put you off. Instead, choose lighter fabrics with a mixture of synthetic materials and cotton, which are designed to deal with moisture better. They don't need to be super-expensive; there are options to suit every budget, but, as always, my advice is to buy the best you can afford.

One other really important element of clothing is layering to keep yourself warm and comfortable. A T-shirt, a thin fleece and a rain- and windproof jacket will provide you with the best way to stay warm on cold winter or autumn days.

BACKPACKS

A must for longer walks or commuting, a good backpack is worth the investment. It's also worth buying from an outdoors store with really knowledgeable staff. Using a backpack that's right for you will be more comfortable and put less pressure on your back and core and even your glutes. Personally, I would recommend one with both chest and waist straps, which take the weight of the backpack and make your walk much more enjoyable.

WEIGHTED VESTS

Weighted vests have been around for a long time but have become really common in the last year or so. A weighted vest is just what it says – a vest with weights in it that makes the walk harder. A simpler version is a backpack with something heavy in it, like a bag of potatoes or some water bottles. Both options help to improve the benefits of a walk as you have to work harder to keep the same pace, especially if it is a hilly route. That's great for your lungs and your muscles, but just be careful if you have back issues as the extra weight can put strain on your back.

TECHNOLOGY AND WALKING

A walk can be really simple and basic – that's one of the best things about it – but you can use technology to make your walk more challenging, more enjoyable and more beneficial to your health. Here are some of the ways that technology can improve your walk.

GPS WATCH

A GPS watch is one of the more expensive investments, but if you are a year-round walker or using walking to really improve your health, it's a very, very handy piece of kit. They range in price from €150 to €800 and for most people, myself included, the low- to mid-range watches are the ones to buy. A GPS watch measures your speed, distance, calories used and heart rate. Most upload the content to an app on your phone via Bluetooth. If you are competitive or like charting your progress, this is essential kit. You can see yourself progress as you get fitter and faster. A GPS watch will also keep track of your routes and lots more. There are no specific brands to recommend as the quality of these watches is generally so good.

BLUETOOTH HEADPHONES

Many people like to listen to music, an audio book or a podcast, or have a chat with a friend while they are walking. It passes the time, encourages you to get out and get moving and for many people it can make a huge difference. You have a few options in terms of what headphones to use. The current trend is the large ear-covering headphones, but they get sweaty, uncomfortable and really cumbersome to wear.

Another option is in-ear wireless headphones, a really good choice. Comfortable, easy to set up and with a good battery life, they are really affordable now too.

My own preference is bone-conduction headphones. These are wireless, and sit just at the front of the ear rather than in the ear. They are really comfortable and the best part is that you can still hear noises around you, such as cars or bikes or people, so they are great for safety too.

APPS

Another really handy option is apps like MapMyRun, MapMyWalk or Strava. There are lots more, but these are my favourites. They record and store your walking routes, details, speed, distances, etc. You can join communities, follow your friends' workouts and track your own. There are paid versions but for most people the free versions are perfect.

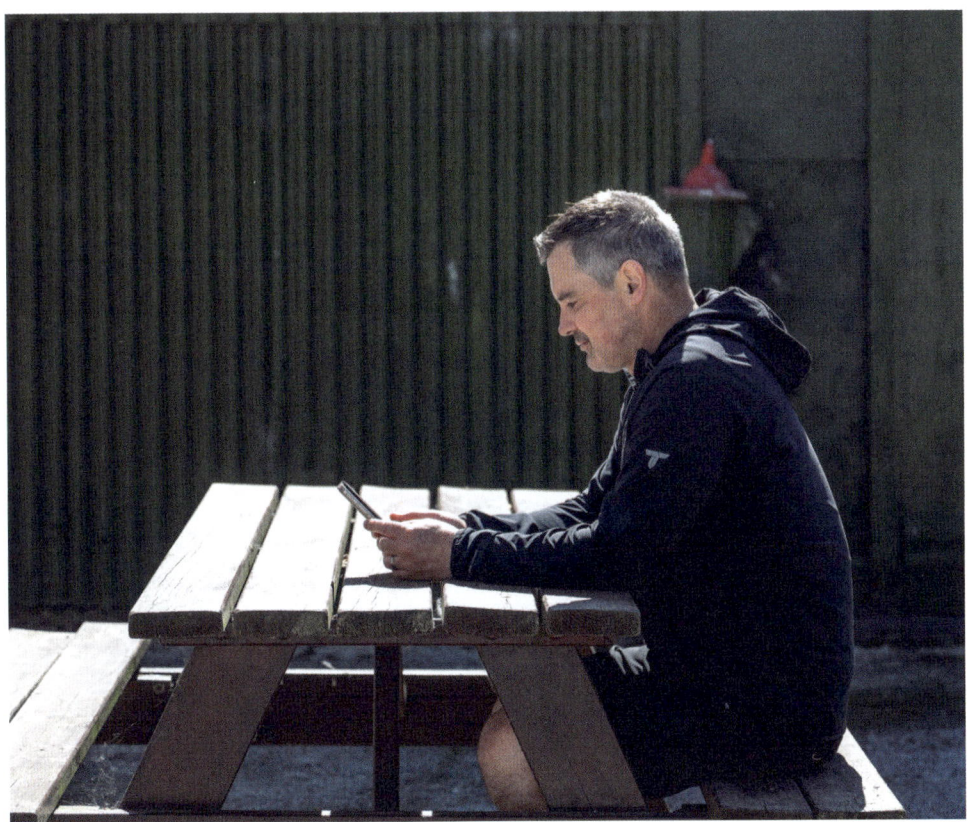

SOME KIT IDEAS FOR DIFFERENT WALKS

SHORT WALK: AN HOUR OR LESS

+ Rain jacket
+ Hat and gloves in winter
+ Small bottle of water
+ Phone, in case you need to make an emergency call

LONG WALK: 1-3 HOURS

+ Rain jacket
+ Hat and gloves in winter
+ Backpack
+ Water and snack (fruit)
+ Compeed blister plasters and Vaseline
+ Phone, in case you need to make an emergency call

VERY LONG WALK: 3 HOURS OR MORE

+ Rain jacket
+ Hat and gloves in winter
+ Backpack
+ Water and snacks (fruit) and sandwich or wrap
+ Compeed plasters and Vaseline
+ Phone, in case you need to make an emergency call
+ Spare socks in case yours get wet

REDUCING THE RISK OF BLISTERS AND CHAFING

Blisters and chafing are two things that really make a walk miserable and often put people off starting or continuing. The good news is that with some simple tips you can reduce the risk of getting them.

First, your clothing and runners are key. Having shoes or runners that fit properly means your feet won't rub against the insides of them. If you have really soft feet, walking around the house barefoot is a simple way to toughen up your feet really fast. Next up, apply Vaseline to any areas where you normally get blisters or chafing, such as between your toes, the outsides of your feet, around your nipples, the insides of your legs or under your arms. If you're doing a long walk, bring more with you just in case.

If you get a blister on your walk, Compeed plasters will fix the issue straight away. They are so handy and I always have some with me on a long walk.

After a walk, steeping your feet in Epsom salts can be a great way to ease any pain, clean them properly and help them to recover too.

RECOVERING FROM A HARD WALK

We have all had that muscle soreness from a long or challenging walk, so here are some really simple ways to feel better!

+ *Epsom salts bath:* Epsom salts are cheap and really effective for recovering. Run a hot bath, add a scoop of salts and relax. Some of the fragranced salts are really lovely and you will be amazed at what a big difference they make.
+ *More flexibility work:* The stretches in this book will give you a simple and effective routine to help you recover at the end of your walk, but doing more flexibility work generally will also help. Yoga, tai chi and Pilates are all great ways to stay supple and reduce the risk of injury.
+ *Muscle rubs:* These are great for rubbing on muscular aches and pains. Just make sure you wash your hands afterwards! Deep Heat, Tiger Balm and udder cream are just some of the muscle rubs out there. I use them all the time and find them really effective.

- *Massage:* What's not to love about a good massage? It's a great way to improve your recovery but also to stay well generally. A sports or deep tissue massage will have you feeling like new. Another option is a massage gun, which is something we use with clients all the time. It's great for home use and it will make a big difference to your recovery.
- *Nutrition:* When you exercise, you put your muscles under pressure and create microtears in the muscle fibres. These grow back stronger and firmer as part of your recovery, and this is why nutrition is so important. Directly after your walk or hike, you should be aiming to take in some protein and carbohydrates. A flavoured milk is a great option. Then, within 90 minutes, have a meal, with protein, carbohydrates and plenty of colour on the plate.

SUN HEALTH

One aspect of health we tend not to think about in relation to walking is sun and skin health. As someone with a history of melanoma, as I have got older this has become a vital part of my walking. There are two important ways of protecting your body when you're walking in the sun:

1 Get a really good sun cream with a high protection number. I use factor 100, but for most people 50+ will do. On longer walks, remember to reapply it every two hours.
2 Cover up! I use a Tilley sunhat, which is a great way of protecting my face and neck from the sun. I also wear long sleeves and sometimes long lightweight trousers to protect my arms and legs.

If you have any concerns about any moles on your skin, please go to your GP and get them checked.

NUTRITION AND HYDRATION

Now it is time to delve into food – for walking, for wellness and for life. Food is fuel and if you want to feel better, walk better and be healthier you need to ensure that you are fuelling your body in the best way.

I genuinely believe that people don't know what to eat any more. It has become so confusing. I want to make it simple so that you can make small but easy changes to your food.

In general, eating more foods that have fewer ingredients on the label, foods that you have to cook and prep yourself and foods with a short shelf life are three key principles that will transform how you eat. Something I often say to my clients is that we should all try to eat like people used to in the 1950s, when we ate more food that was cooked from scratch and had fewer preservatives in it. There is so much noise at the moment around ultra-processed food, and some of it is so over the top. We all eat some foods that are processed, and that's okay. Everything in moderation.

FOODS BEFORE AND AFTER WALKS

Most walks don't require specific fuelling from a food perspective. If we're eating a normal healthy diet we have enough energy in our muscles to keep us going. But longer hikes and very long walks, such as those in the marathon training plan, are a little different.

If you are going on a long hike or really long training walk, you need to eat a slow-release carbohydrate meal two to three hours beforehand. Porridge, bread, rice and pasta are all perfect options. I prefer the brown/wholegrain varieties as they are slow-release carbohydrates and will give you lots of energy. Add some protein, such as nuts or seeds for your porridge, or chicken, fish, meat, quinoa or lentils for lunch or dinner.

When you're on a long hike or walk you should aim to fuel up every 60 minutes or so. Small, regular snacks are a great way to keep your energy levels up.

Some simple snack options are:

+ Fruit
+ Flapjacks (the recipe in this book is great!)
+ Protein balls
+ Rice cakes
+ Hummus and veg
+ Half a small sandwich.

Along with your snacks, you should aim to drink 200–300ml of fluid per hour. If the day is really hot or you are walking somewhere like the Camino in the summer, some electrolytes are handy to have too during one of your stops.

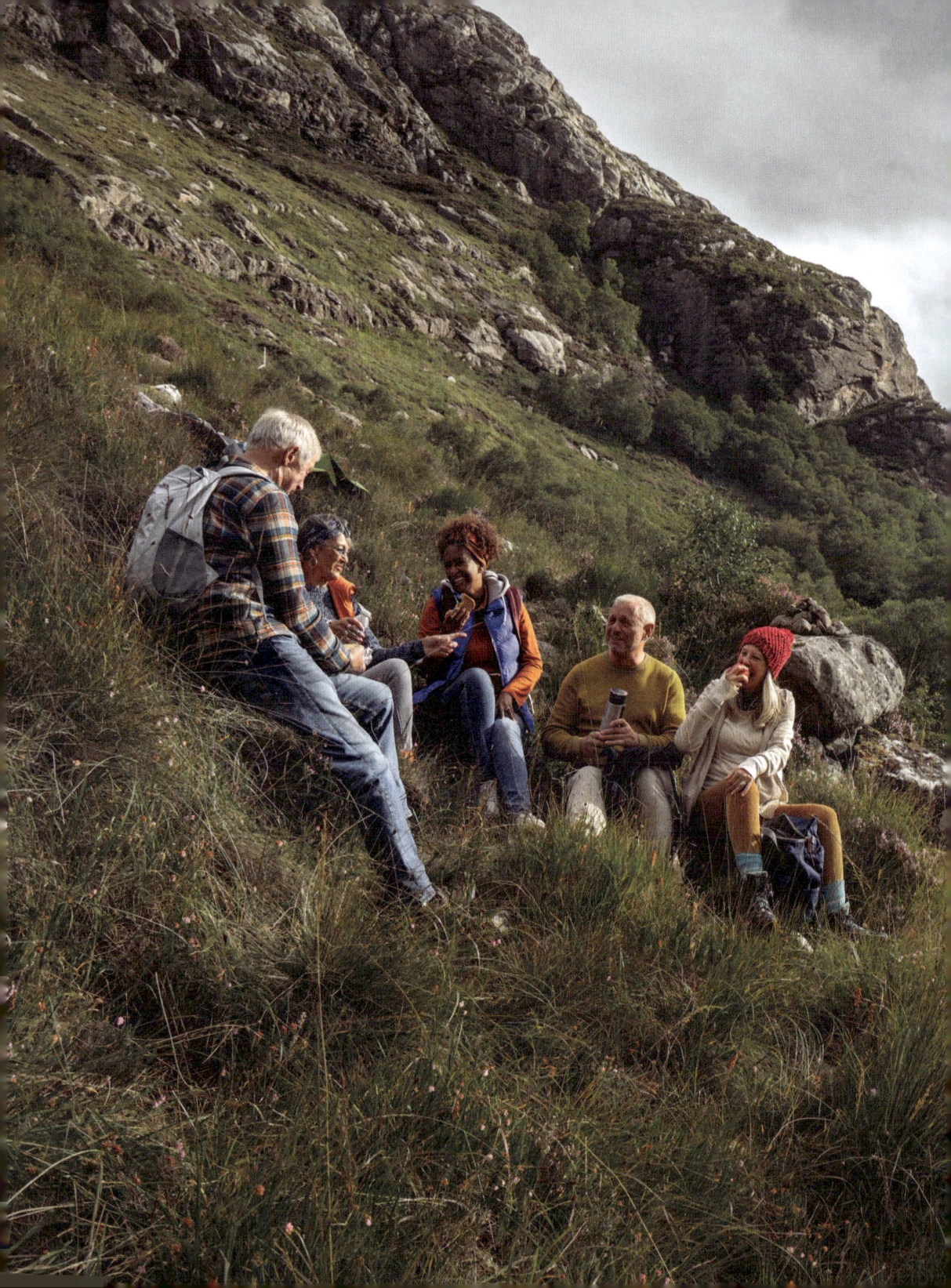

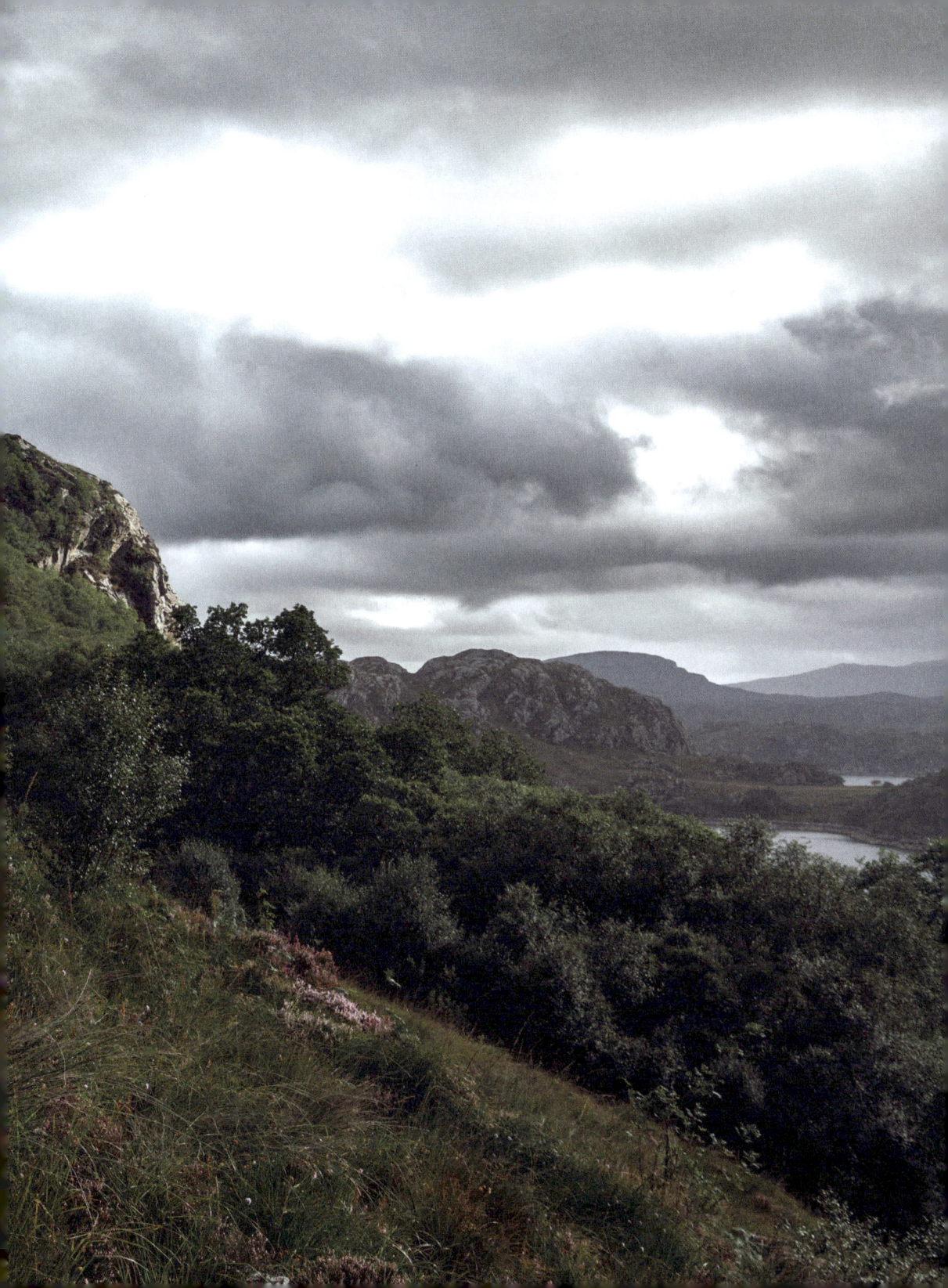

RECIPES

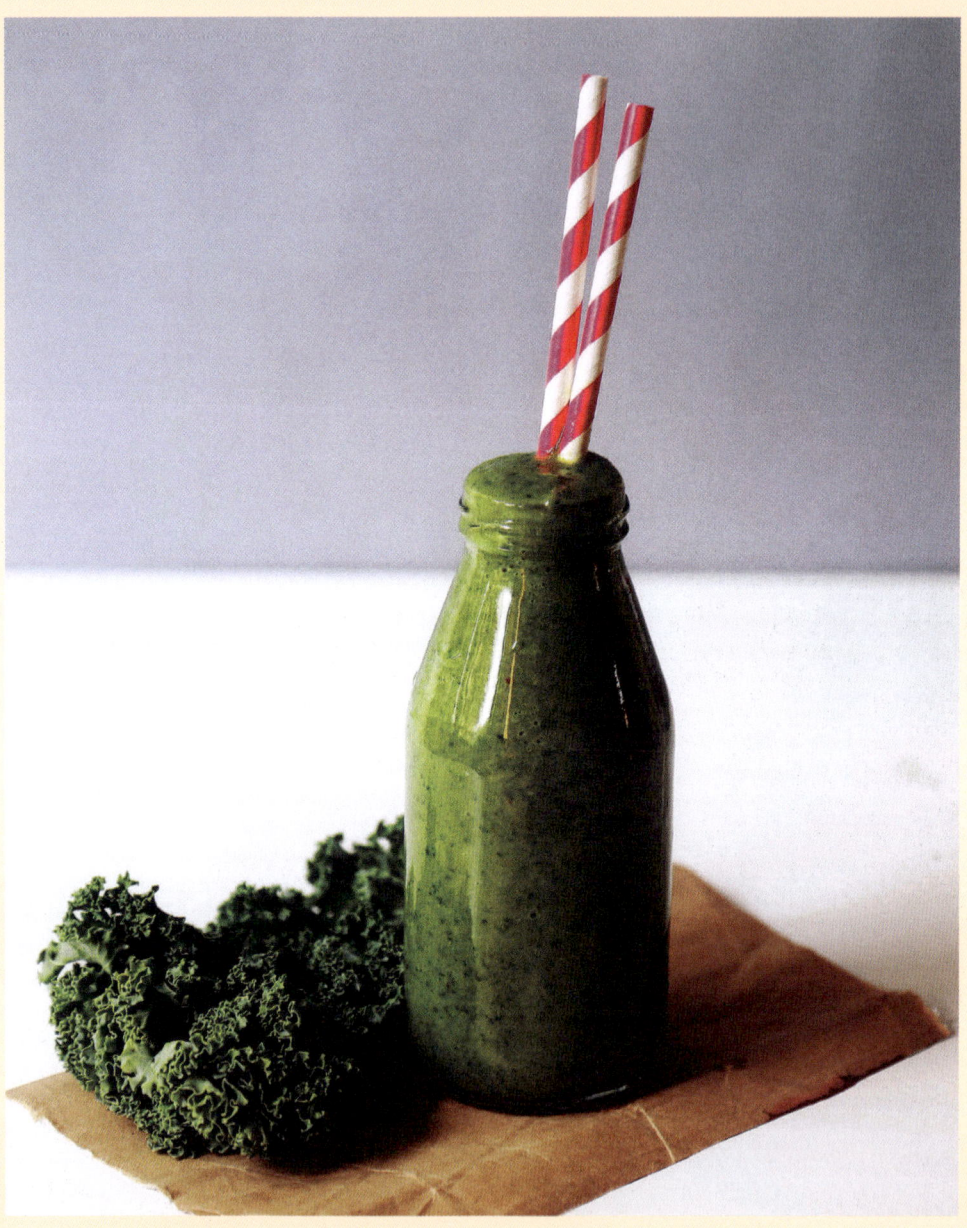

BREAKFAST SMOOTHIE

This is super quick and nutritious. If, like me, you are always rushing in the morning and need something quick and healthy, try this for size.

SERVES: 1

WHAT YOU NEED

100ml milk or dairy-free alternative

1 ripe pear, cored

1 small apple, cored

1 handful of kale

2 tbsp organic jumbo porridge oats

a thumb-sized piece of ginger, peeled and chopped

½ tsp honey

HOW TO MAKE IT

1 It couldn't be easier! Simply put all the ingredients in a blender and blend.
2 You could also add a scoop of protein powder if you like. Aim for one with low sugar content – remember, 4g of sugar is the equivalent of a teaspoon.

BERRIES WITH LOW-FAT YOGHURT AND TOASTED OATS

Here is another simple option I bring on morning hikes if I am out early.

SERVES: 1

WHAT YOU NEED

Handful of fresh berries, such as blueberries and strawberries

2 tbsp porridge oats

2 tbsp low-fat yoghurt

HOW TO MAKE IT

1 Heat a dry frying pan and place the oats in the pan. Toast for 5–7 minutes on a medium heat until they are golden brown.

2 Allow the oats to cool, then mix with the berries and the yoghurt and pop them into a container.

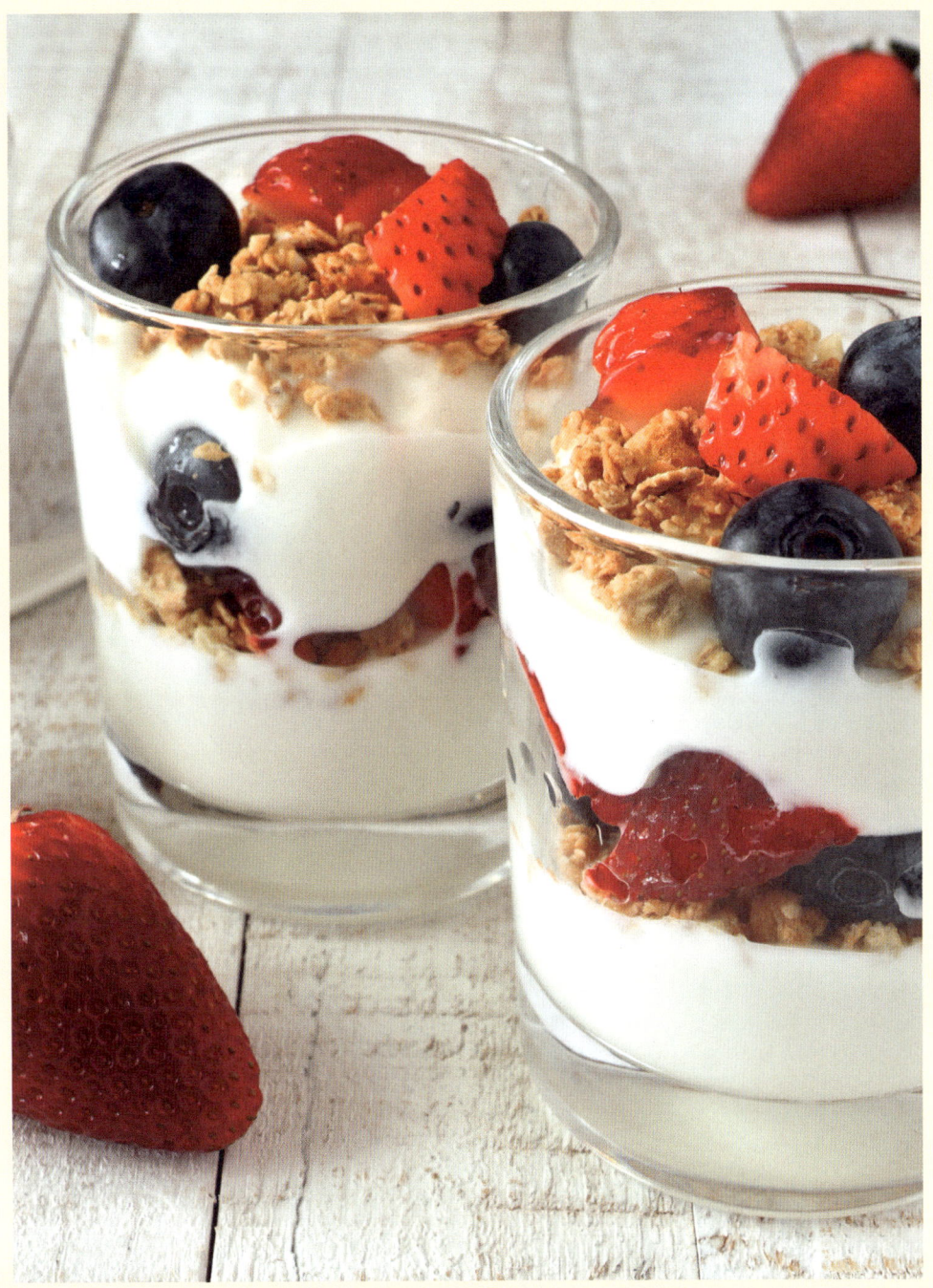

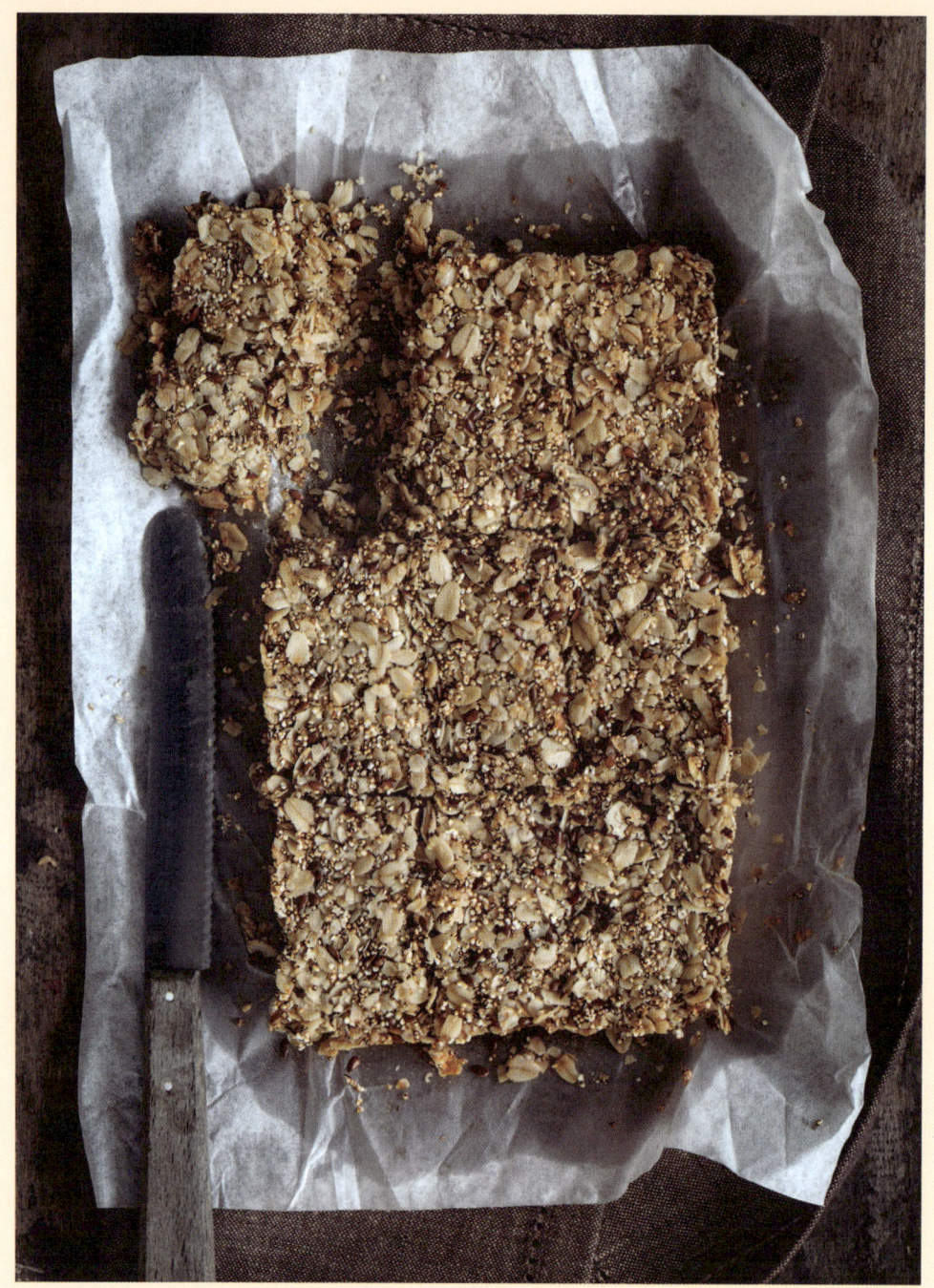

FLAPJACKS

These are a really handy snack to take on a hillwalk or a long walk. Easy to make, they last for ages and will give you lots of energy.

MAKES: 10 FLAPJACKS

WHAT YOU NEED

110g porridge oats

100g nuts of your choice, roughly chopped

75g dates, roughly chopped

50g dried apricots, roughly chopped

1 tbsp rapeseed oil

100g honey

HOW TO MAKE THEM

1 Preheat the oven to 160°C/140°C Fan/325°F/gas mark 3.

2 Line a 20cm square baking tin with baking parchment.

3 Mix the oats, nuts, dates and apricots together in a large bowl. Then add the oil and honey and mix thoroughly.

4 Transfer the mixture to the baking tin, spread evenly and flatten firmly using the back of a spoon.

5 Bake for 20 minutes.

6 Remove from the oven and score into 10 rectangles while still warm.

7 Allow to cool completely, then turn out of the tin and break into 10 individual flapjacks. Store in an airtight container in a cool place. They will keep for 10 days or so.

PROTEIN BALLS

Super trendy and super handy, these supply a good protein hit and provide lots of energy too.

MAKES: 15 BALLS

WHAT YOU NEED

150g porridge oats

50g protein powder of your choice (I use vanilla whey)

1 tbsp ground flaxseeds

pinch of ground cinnamon

2 tbsp maple syrup

1 tsp vanilla extract

150g nut butter of your choice (I use peanut)

4 tbsp plant milk

25g chocolate chips

HOW TO MAKE THEM

1 Combine the oats, protein powder, flaxseeds and cinnamon in a large bowl.
2 Add the maple syrup, vanilla extract, nut butter, milk and chocolate chips and stir well to combine.
3 Using damp hands, roll the mixture into 15 balls (they should be about 30g each). Arrange on a plate and chill for 30 minutes until firm.

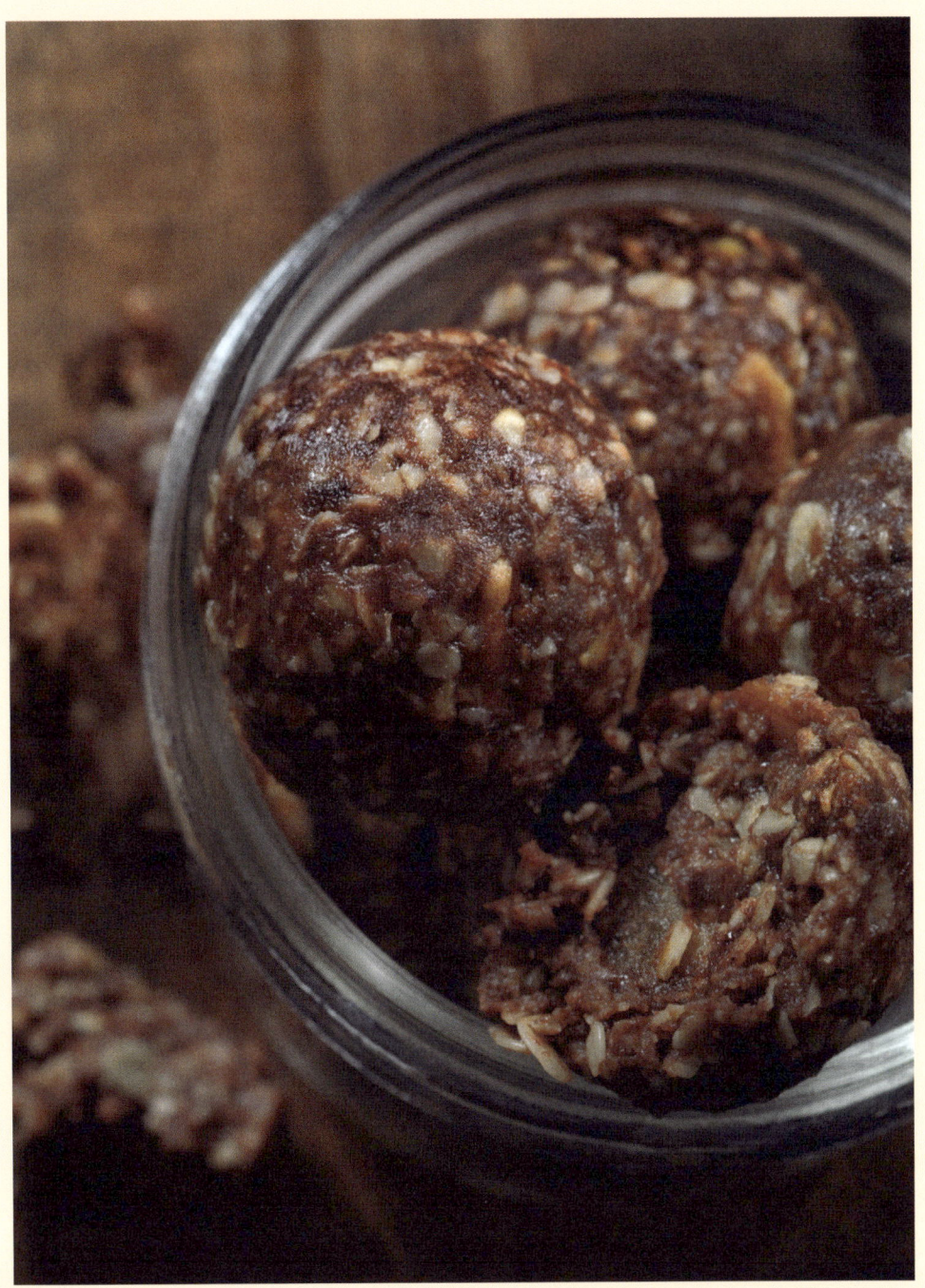

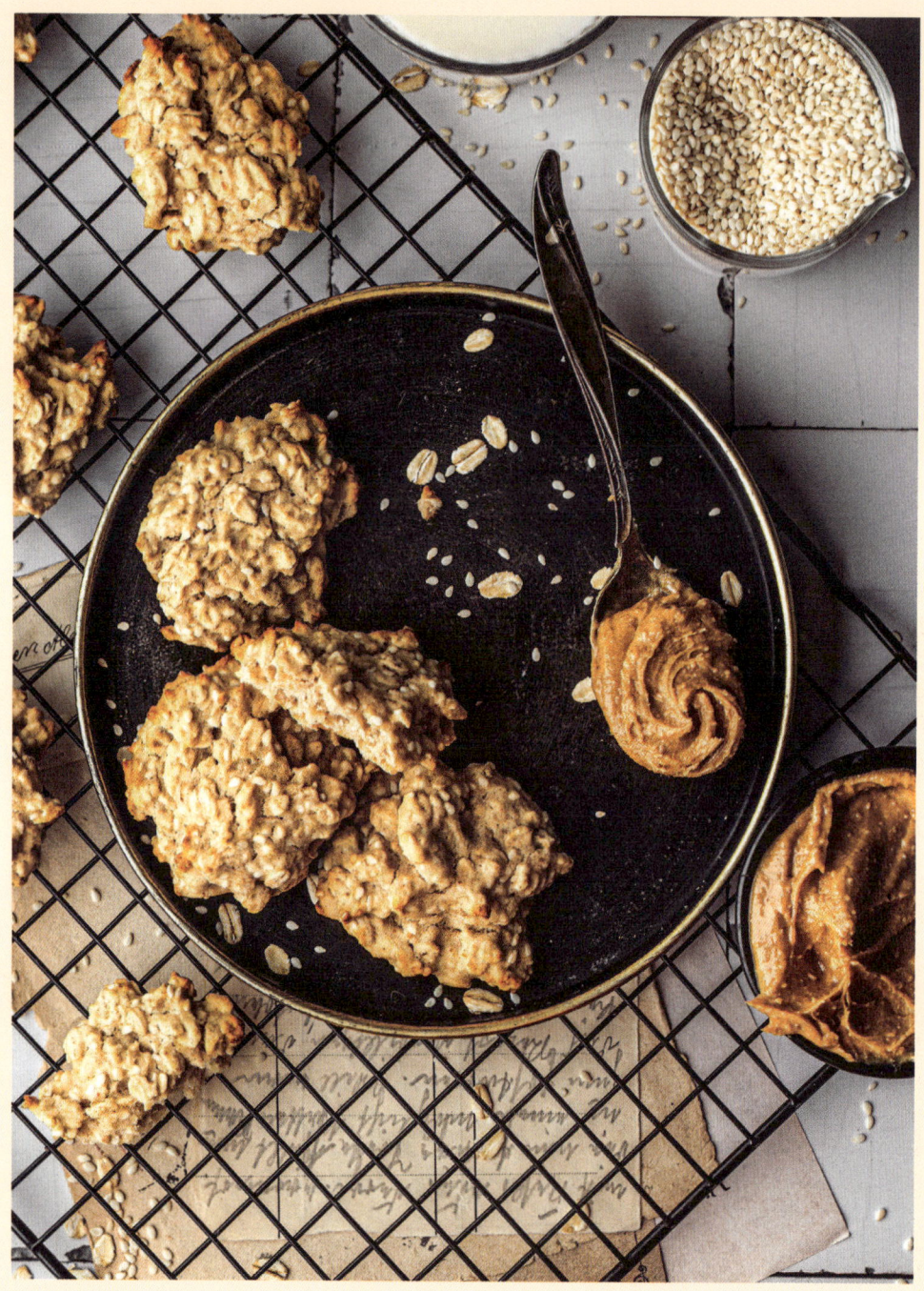

PEANUT BUTTER AND OAT COOKIES

Peanut butter is certainly in fashion at the moment, so I thought I would give you a recipe for peanut butter and oat cookies. They're delicious and actually quite healthy.

MAKES: 6–8

WHAT YOU NEED

170g honey

50g coconut oil

20g unsweetened cocoa powder

125g crunchy peanut butter

65g rolled oats

85g unsweetened shredded coconut

2 tbsp flaxseeds

HOW TO MAKE THEM

1 Combine the honey, coconut oil and cocoa powder in a medium saucepan. Stir over medium heat until the coconut oil is completely melted and the mixture is smooth and warm.

2 Add the peanut butter and stir until completely melted.

3 Turn off the heat and stir in the oats.

4 Cover with a lid for 5 minutes. Remove the lid and add a third of the coconut and all the flaxseeds.

5 Use a spoon to scoop out the cookies and sprinkle each one with some of the remaining coconut.

6 Lightly flatten the cookies with a spatula and repeat this process.

7 Refrigerate the cookies until they are completely chilled.

SIMPLE SPORTS DRINK

This is really easy to make and it's a healthier version of what you might buy in a shop, since it uses real lemon or lime juice rather than artificial flavouring.

MAKES: 500ML

WHAT YOU NEED

500ml cold water

1 heaped tbsp sugar

Juice of a whole lemon or lime

Pinch of salt

HOW TO MAKE IT

1   Simply mix all the ingredients together, give it a good shake and chill!

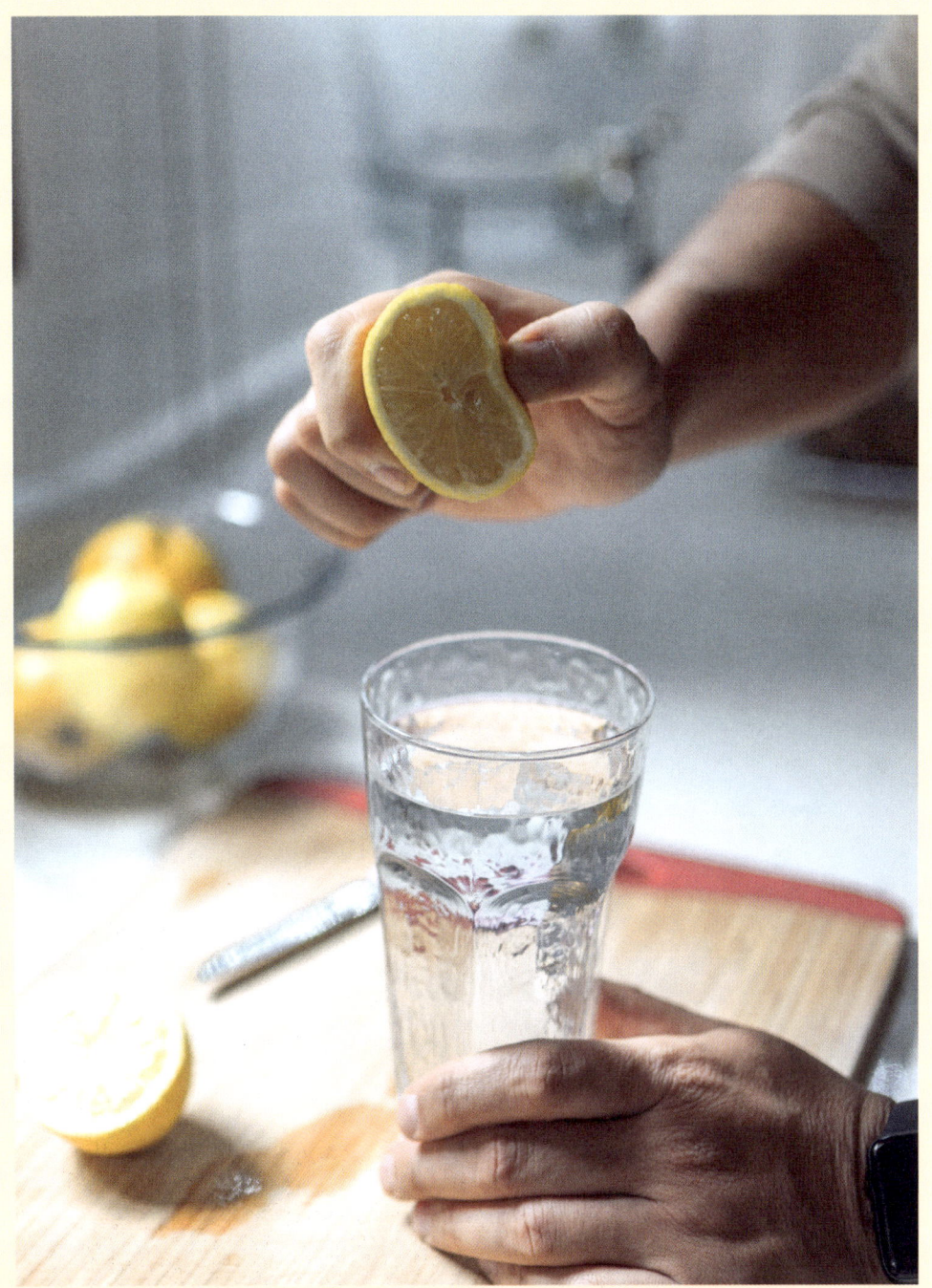

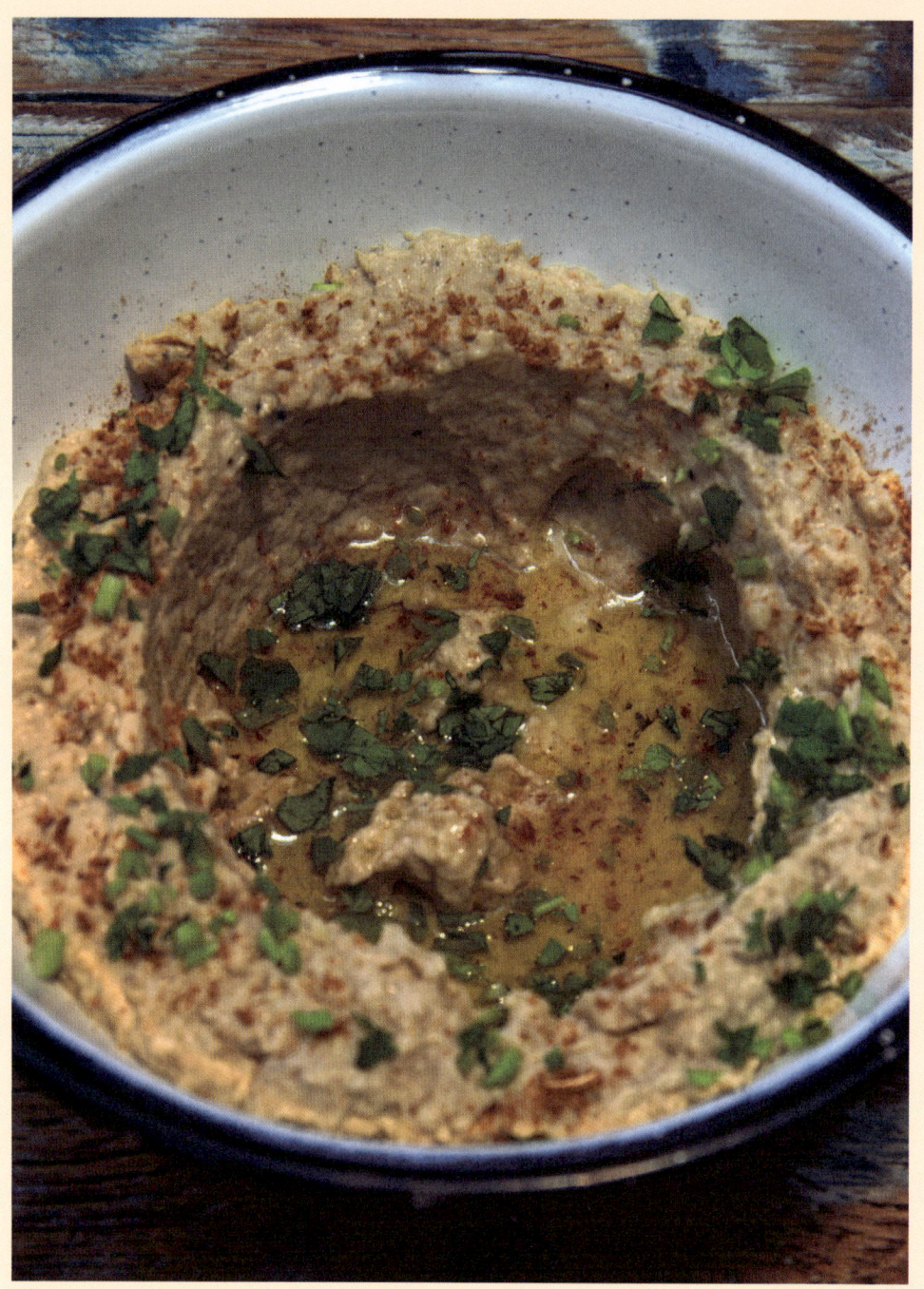

Dips and vegetables or pittas/tortillas are great snacks to bring on a hike. Here are two of my favourite dips. Serve them with cucumber, carrot or pepper batons, olives, cherry tomatoes …

BABA GANOUSH

SERVES: 6

WHAT YOU NEED

3 large aubergines

2 cloves of garlic, peeled and chopped

1 lemon, juiced

3 tsp tahini paste

4 tbsp olive oil

HOW TO MAKE IT

1 Preheat the oven to 180°C/350°F/gas mark 4.
2 Prick the skins of the aubergines all over with a fork and put them in the oven for around 45 minutes until the skin is collapsing (this gives them a smoky flavour). Take out of the oven, allow to cool a little and scrape out the flesh. Discard the skins.
3 Put the aubergine flesh in a blender and add the other ingredients. Blend to a paste. Alternatively, you could put all the ingredients into a bowl and whisk until they form a paste.
4 Serve with wholemeal pitta or vegetables.

HUMMUS

WHAT YOU NEED

225g tin of chickpeas, drained

Juice of ½ lemon

2 tbsp tahini paste

½ tsp ground cumin

1 clove of garlic, peeled and chopped

HOW TO MAKE IT

1 Purée the drained chickpeas with the lemon juice, tahini, cumin, garlic and a little water to loosen the mix.

2 Serve with toasted brown pitta, halved cherry tomatoes, pepper and cucumber batons and some black olives.

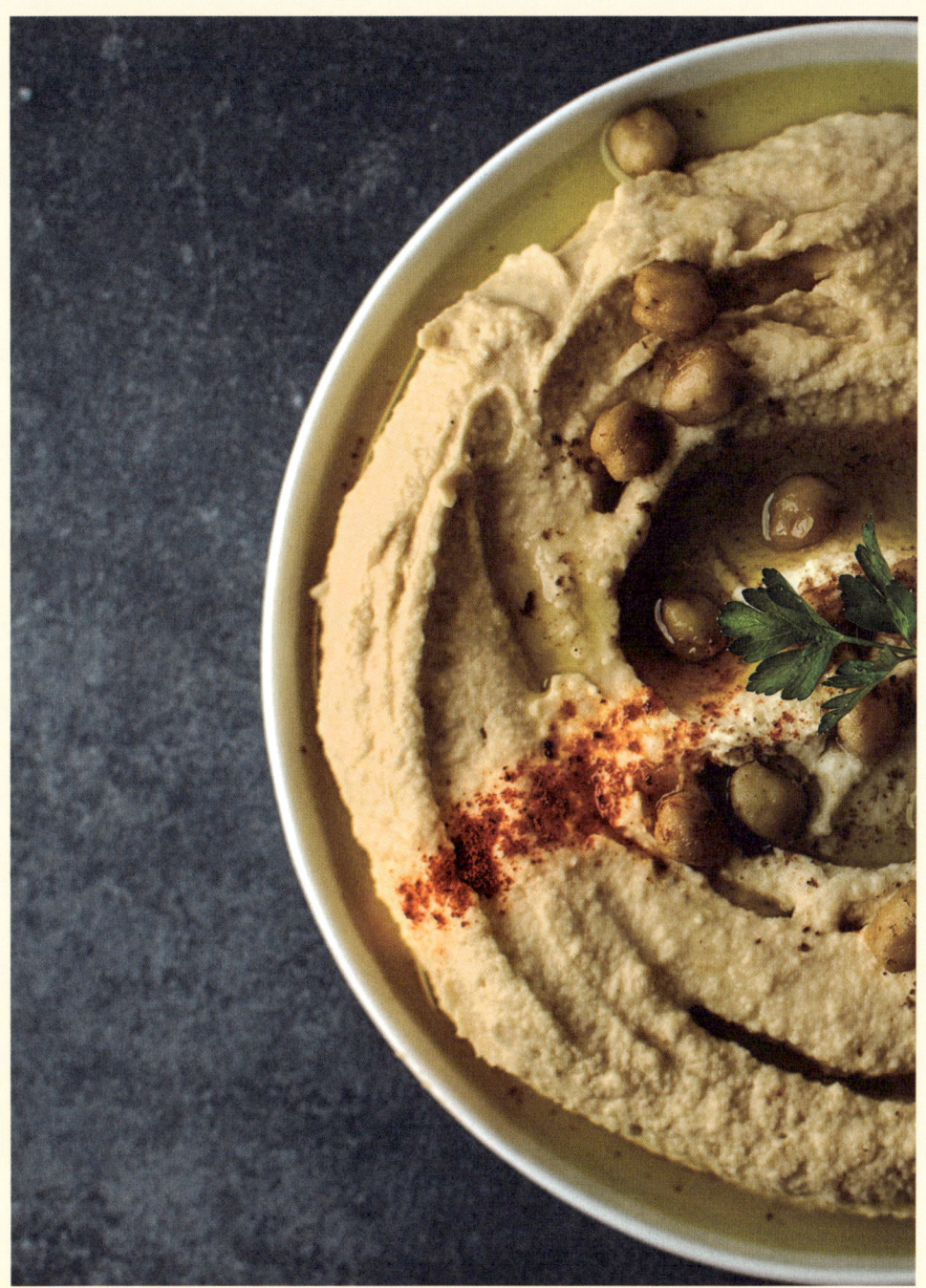

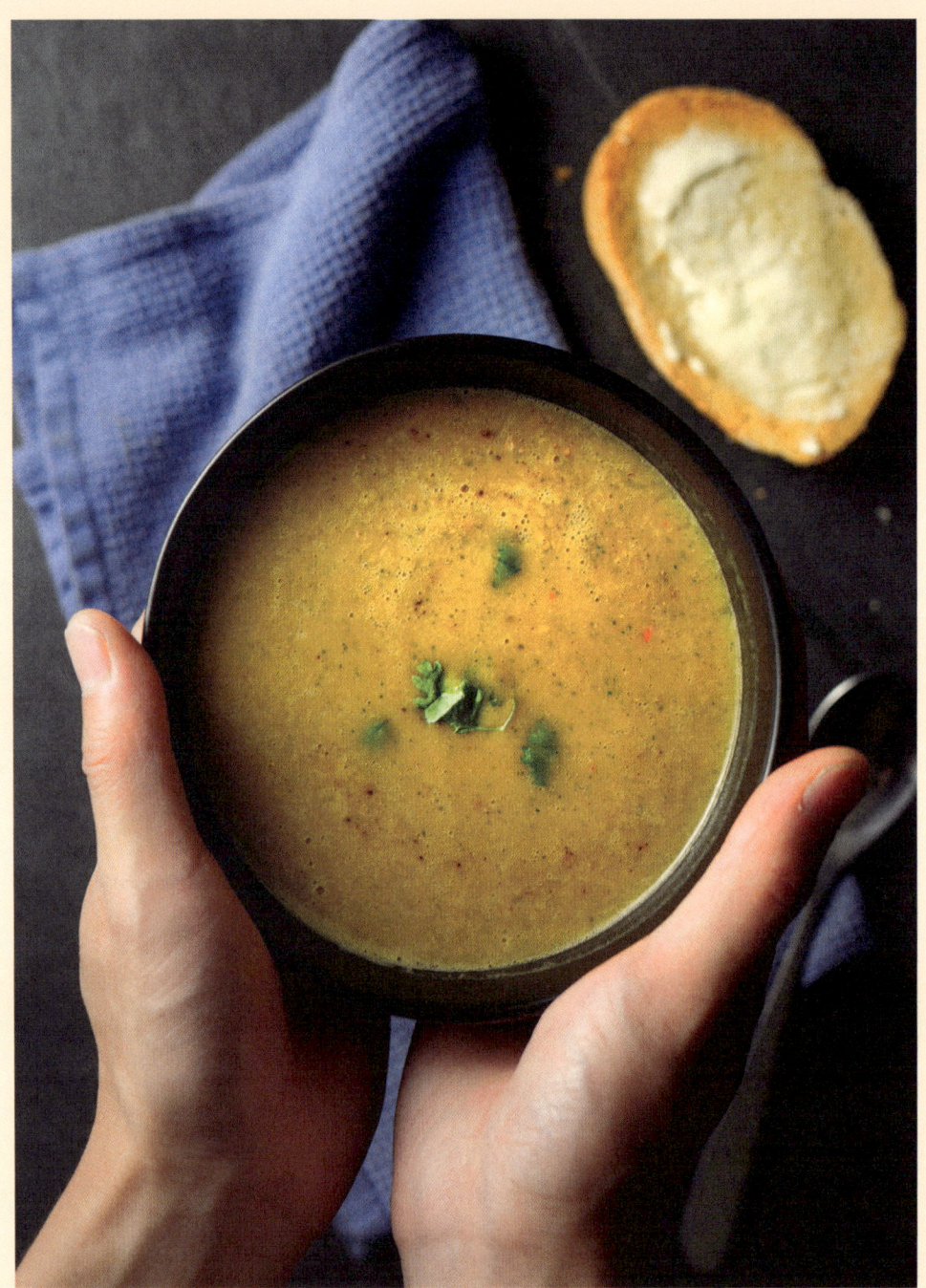

SIMPLE SUPERFOOD SOUP

As I have got older I've got into the habit of bringing a flask of soup with me on long walks. It's so handy and a total game-changer!

SERVES: 4

WHAT YOU NEED

400g tin kidney beans, cannellini beans, butter beans or chickpeas, rinsed and drained

2 medium to large carrots, sliced

3 medium broccoli florets

1 large onion, diced

1 red pepper, sliced

1 yellow pepper, sliced

2 cloves garlic, minced or thinly sliced

2 medium sweet potatoes, diced

½ tsp chopped or dried basil

½ tsp chopped or dried oregano

1–2 bay leaves

1 tbsp soy sauce

Freshly ground black pepper to taste

2 organic vegetable stock cubes

HOW TO MAKE IT

1 Put all the ingredients in a saucepan with a litre of boiling water and simmer until the vegetables are soft.

2 Allow to cool a little, then remove the bay leaves and blend.

3 Don't forget to freeze the leftovers!

VEGETABLE SOUP

WHAT YOU NEED

1 tbsp olive oil

1 onion, peeled and chopped

1 clove of garlic, chopped

1 courgette, chopped

2 peppers, chopped

2 carrots, chopped

Handful of broccoli florets

Handful of green beans

Handful of shredded cabbage or spinach

4 sticks of celery

2 x 400g tins chopped tomatoes

1l chicken or vegetable stock

A few drops of Tabasco or 1–2 fresh chillies, chopped (optional)

HOW TO MAKE IT

1 Fry the onion in the olive oil for 3–4 minutes until softened.

2 Add the garlic and the remaining fresh vegetables, which should be in even-sized chunks. Cook for a few minutes, then add the tinned tomatoes and the stock, and the chilli or Tabasco if using.

3 Simmer for about 15 minutes or until the vegetables are tender.

4 You can either purée the soup or leave it chunky.

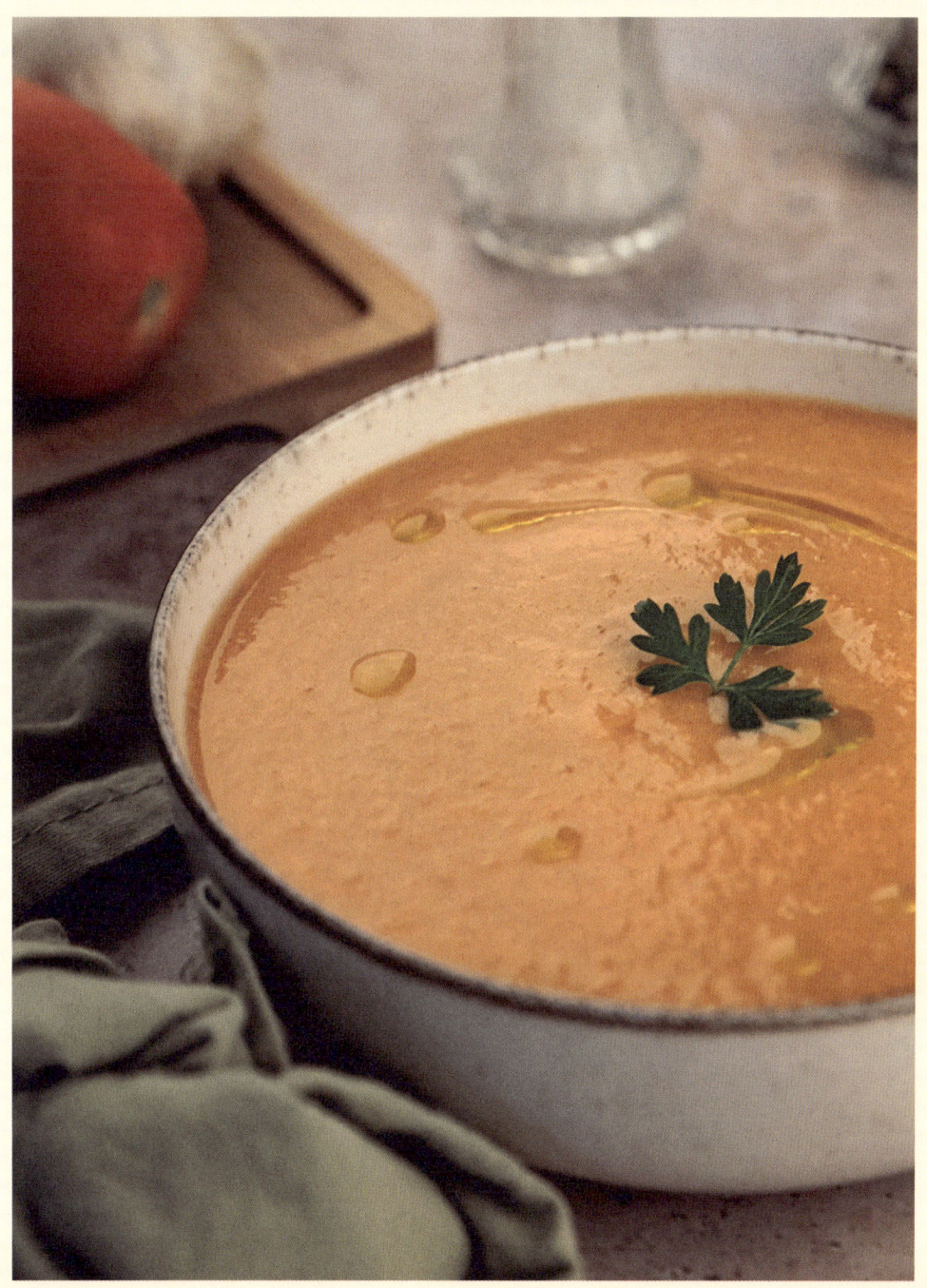

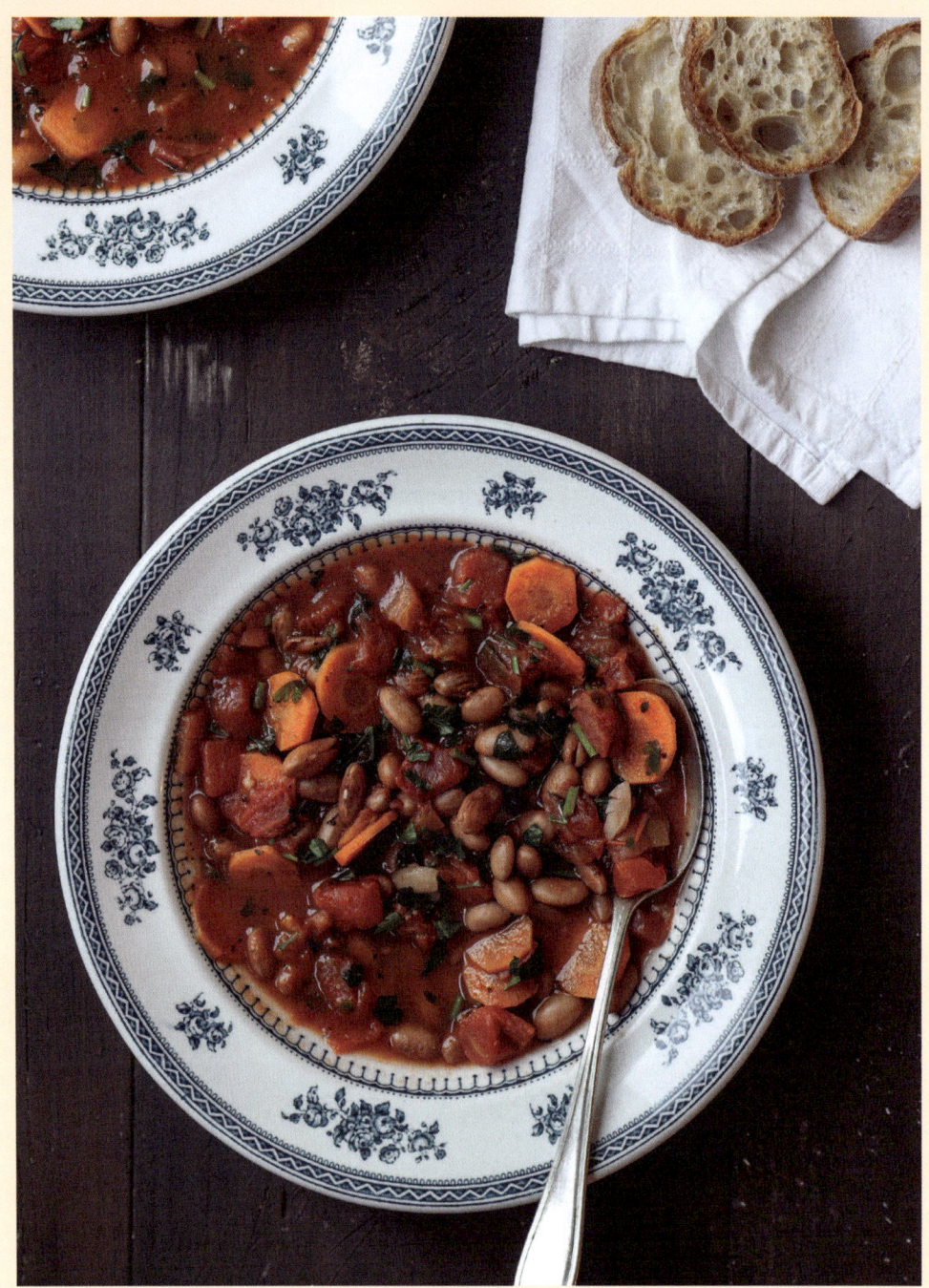

TOMATO AND BEAN SOUP

SERVES: 6

WHAT YOU NEED

2 tbsp coconut oil

2 medium onions, diced

4 cloves of garlic, crushed

400g tin chopped tomatoes

2 medium carrots, diced

400g tin kidney beans, rinsed and drained

1.5l good vegetable stock

Freshly ground black pepper

1 tsp dried oregano (even better if you have fresh: 2-3 stalks should be sufficient)

HOW TO MAKE IT

1   It really couldn't be simpler. Put everything in a saucepan, simmer for 15 minutes or so. You can either leave it as it is or blend before serving. If you are using fresh oregano, remove the stalks before blending.

QUINOA AND BROCCOLI SALAD
WITH AVOCADO PESTO

Quinoa is an amazing source of protein and broccoli is one of the most nutritious vegetables there is.

SERVES: 4

WHAT YOU NEED

2 medium heads broccoli, cut into florets

8 cloves garlic, peeled

4 tbsp olive oil, divided

1 ripe avocado

2 tbsp pine nuts

Squeeze of lemon juice (optional)

170g cooked quinoa

HOW TO MAKE IT

1 Preheat the oven to 200°C/400°F/gas mark 6.
2 Mix the broccoli and garlic cloves with 1 tablespoon of the olive oil. Roast for 15 minutes.
3 Set half of the roasted broccoli florets aside for the salad.
4 Now put the rest of the roasted broccoli, the roasted garlic, avocado flesh, pine nuts and 3 tablespoons of olive oil in a blender, and blend to a smooth purée. You can add lemon juice if you'd like.
5 Now simply mix the pesto and the reserved broccoli florets into the cooked quinoa.

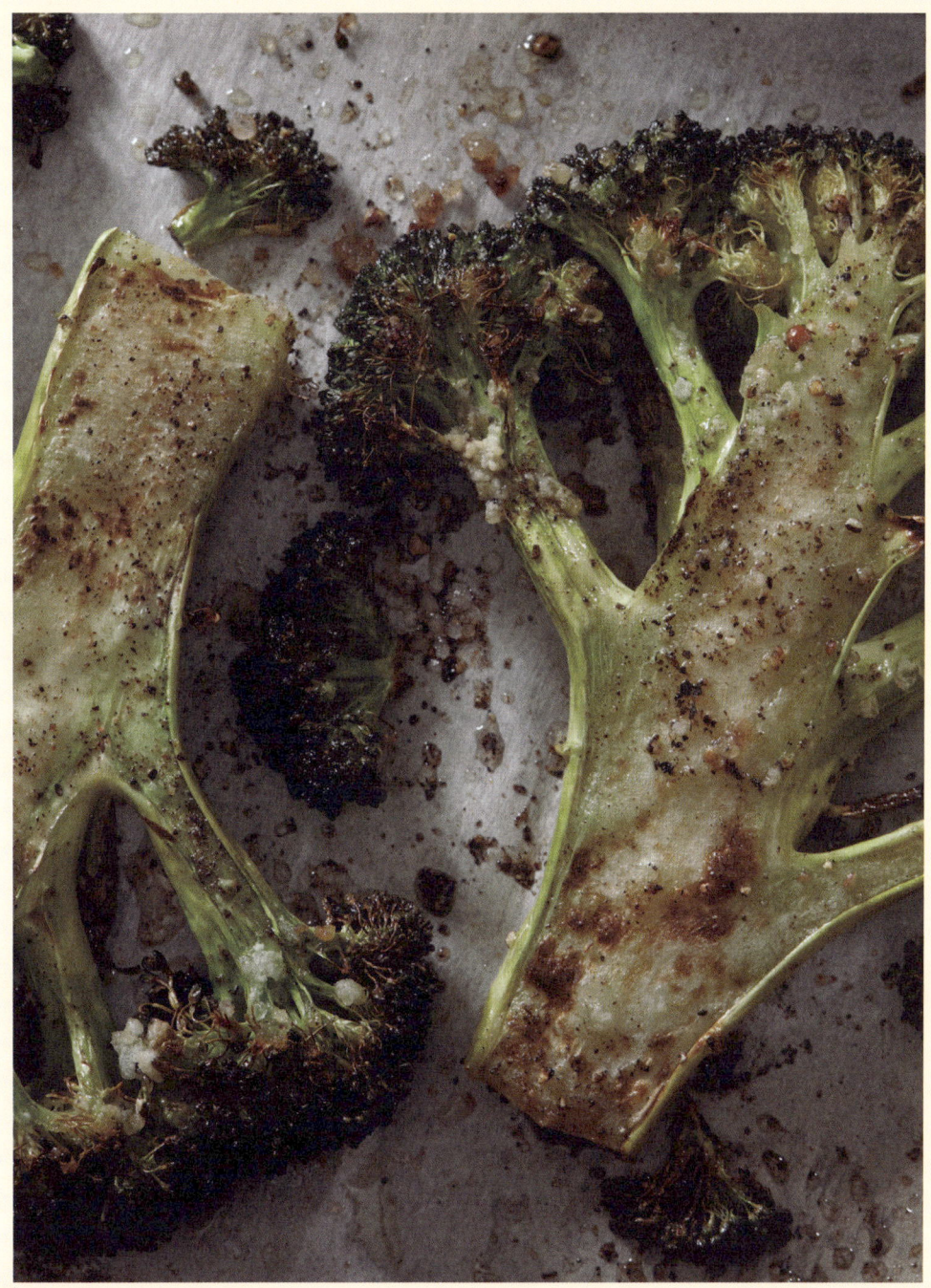

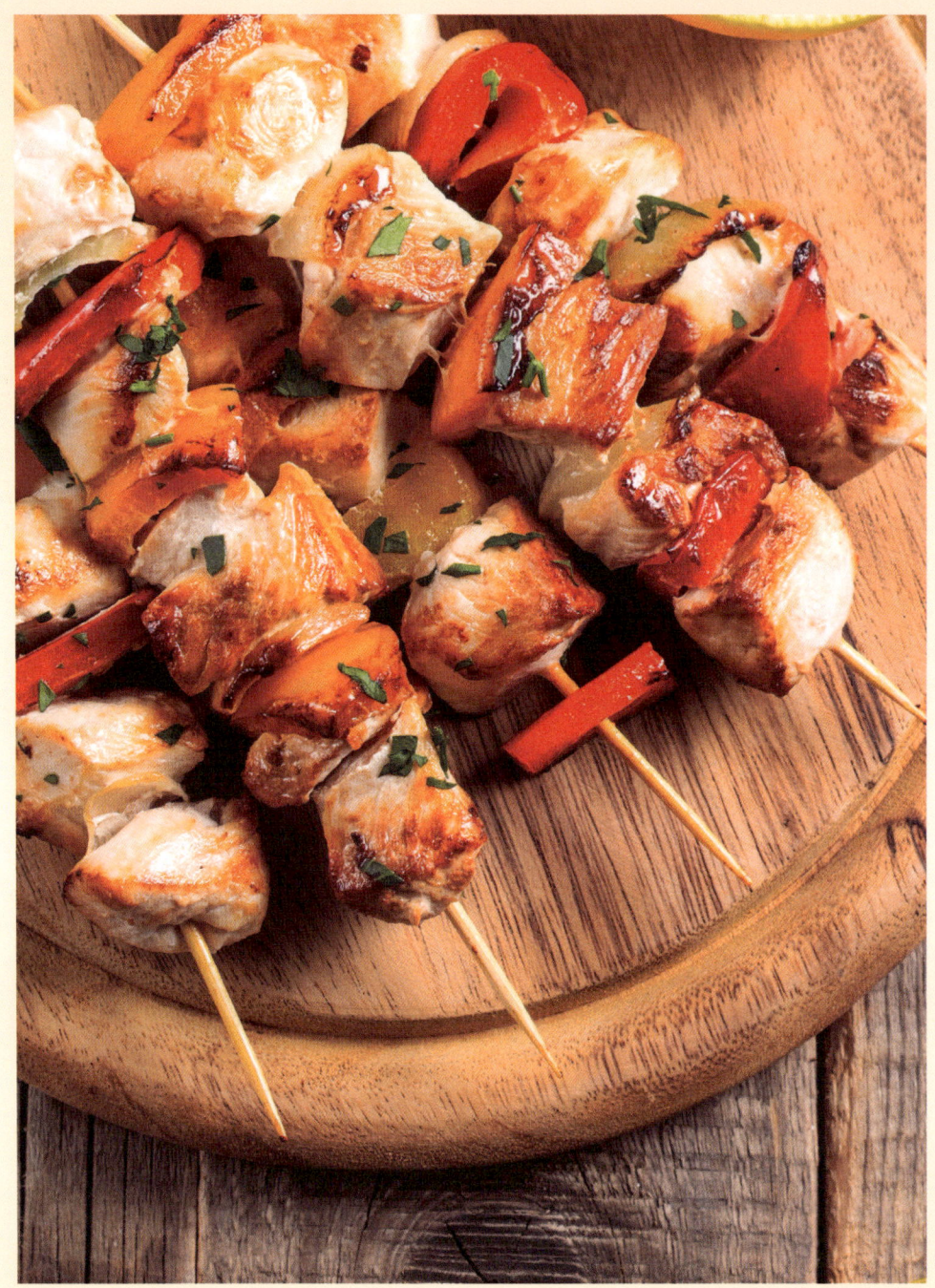

SUPER SIMPLE CHICKEN KEBABS

SERVES: 2

WHAT YOU NEED

Juice of 1 lemon

½ tsp smoked paprika

Small clove (or ½ clove) of garlic, crushed

Ground black pepper

2 chicken fillets

1 red onion

1 red pepper

You'll also need some kebab skewers

HOW TO MAKE IT

1 Mix the lemon juice, paprika, garlic and black pepper. Cut the chicken into bite-sized chunks and marinate in the mixture for 15 minutes.

2 Cut the onion and red pepper into large chunks.

3 Thread the chicken onto the kebab skewers, alternating with the pieces of onion and pepper.

4 Preheat the oven to 180°C/350°F/gas mark 4 and cook the kebabs until cooked through and charred on the outside, approx. 15 minutes.

5 Either eat straight away, or allow to cool and pack them up for a picnic.

TURKEY BURGERS

MAKES: 4 BURGERS

WHAT YOU NEED

300g lean turkey mince

1 onion, finely chopped

1 tsp Tabasco

Pepper

1 egg

Handful of basil, finely chopped

Handful of coriander, finely chopped

HOW TO MAKE IT

1 Mix all the ingredients in a bowl using your hands.

2 Form the mix into burger shapes – you should get four burgers.

3 Preheat the grill to medium and grill the burgers for 10–15 minutes or until cooked through.

4 Serve with a mixed salad or in a burger bun with the usual extras.

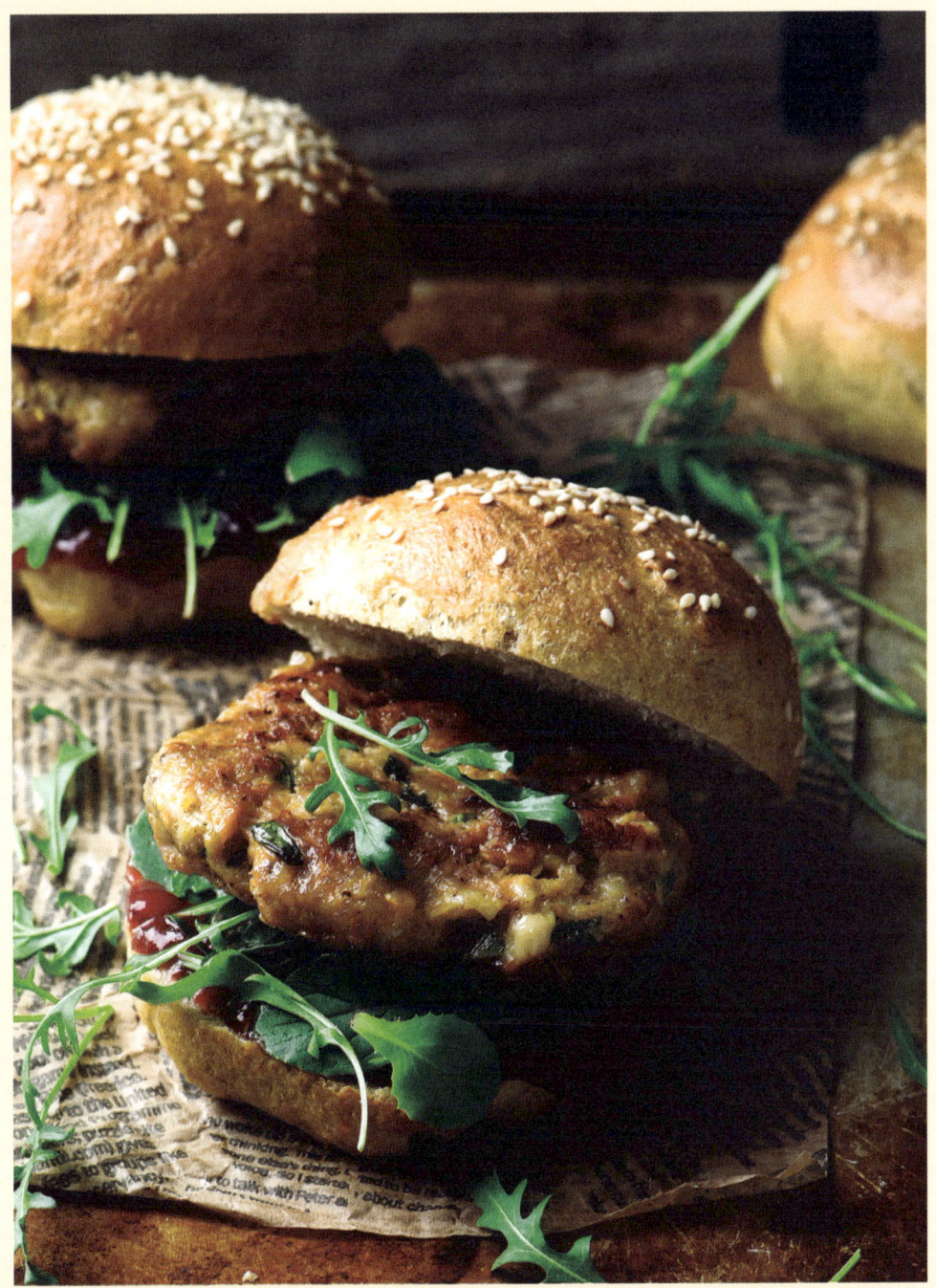

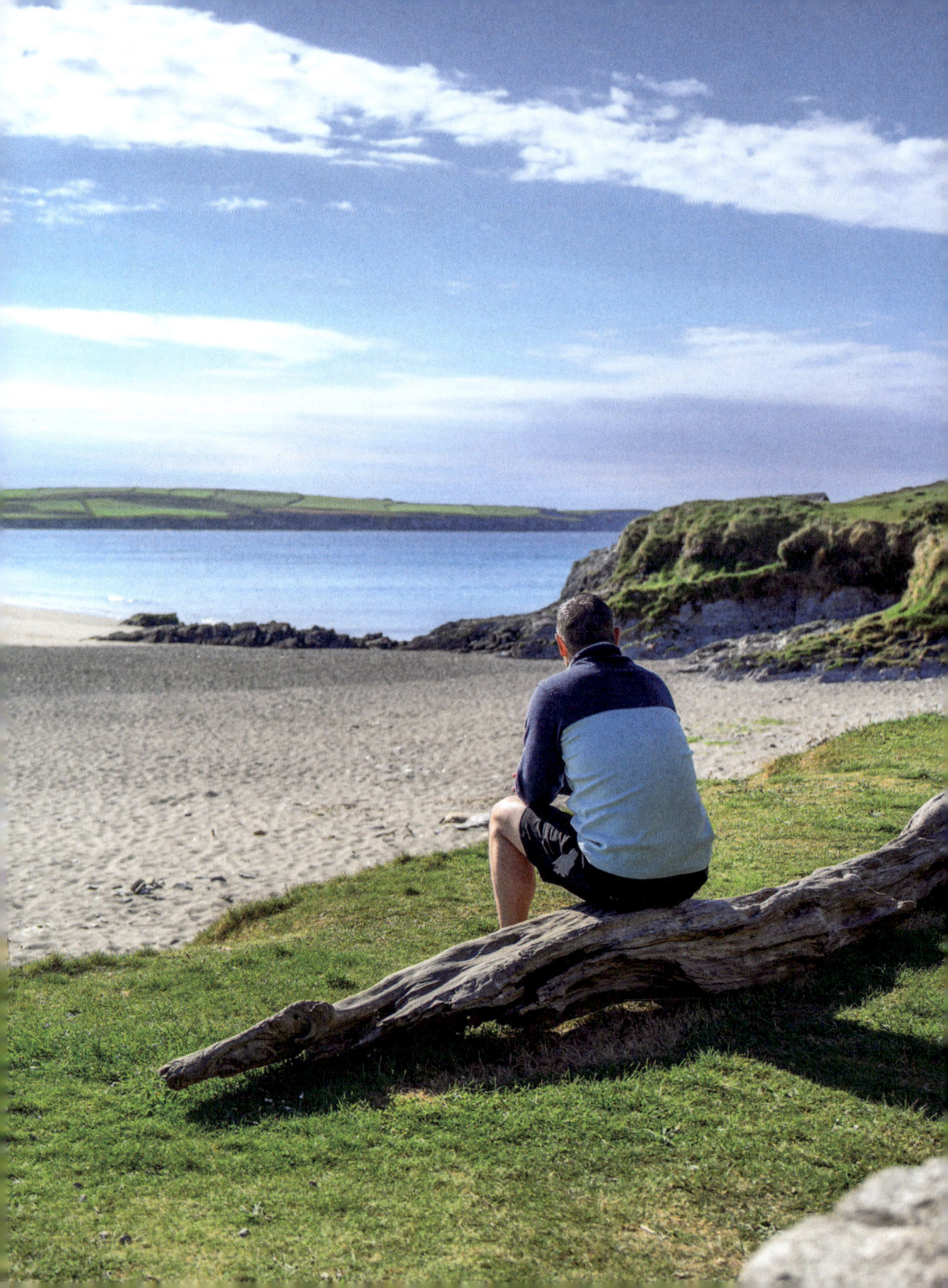

CHAPTER FOUR

NATURE - THE SUPERPOWER YOU DIDN'T KNOW EXISTED

As I'm sure you've realised by now, I think that walking is the most amazing exercise. Any walking is great, but if you are able to walk in nature you will gain even more remarkable benefits. From changing your gut bacteria to reducing your inflammatory markers, increasing serotonin and reducing cortisol, nature is our de-stressing friend. In this chapter I want to bring you into the world of nature and help you realise that you need to get more nature into your life and what that will do for you. You will be amazed by how good adding green and blue to your walks makes you feel. It's a small change you can make to your everyday life.

A study by Nordrum et al. measured the effects of a 1.8km walk in nature and compared it with walking in a built-up environment. It found that spending time in natural environments, like forests, grasslands, gardens and parks, can result in significant mental and physical health benefits, including boosting mood, regulating body temperature, reducing stress, microbiome development, cognitive development, and lower probabilities of cardiovascular disease and diabetes. Isn't that amazing? Spending time in nature not only boosts our mood, it also changes our gut flora. Look again at the range of benefits the researchers report from purely environmental changes. Green exercise (walking in nature) is something we need more and more of.

In 'Doses of neighbourhood nature: The benefits for mental health of living with nature', a study by Cox et al., the researchers found that even low levels of key components of what they call neighbourhood nature can be associated with better mental health, providing promise for preventive health approaches. More and more research is showing us that nature and walking combined can be a superpower for the body and the mind!

THE POWER OF LIGHT AND GETTING OUTSIDE

We know that just being outside improves our health and wellness. I know myself how my mood can be transformed by just stepping outside into the garden, or taking a short walk around the fields near our house. But now we also know that the science backs this up. Green zoning (surrounding yourself with more plants and trees) and blue zoning (surrounding yourself with water and the sky) are nature's natural superpowers. The environment around us has such a profound impact on our health. Surrounding ourselves with nature or making a conscious decision to be in it as much as possible can transform us.

How we live now, in cities and in offices and working all day, we are placing ourselves in an environment that stresses us out and overwhelms us. It's literally burning us out. I have spent 25 years working in health and wellness and I am lucky enough to travel to give talks to companies and work with them to develop corporate wellness programmes. I am always blown away by the differences in how companies create office spaces. Some spaces empower you to work and feel better, with views of nature and lots of natural light. Some are dark and dreary and a much tougher place to work in. More green zones and blue zones in our workplaces would help us to improve how we work, think, interact, deal with stress and lots more.

Studies have shown that our minds and bodies relax in a natural setting. Think about the space you work in. How is it set up? Does it get enough light? If not, how can you get more light in? Can you bring the outside in by adding plants? Can you get outside to walk more? Nature can provide a mental break by allowing us to temporarily escape the demands of everyday life and the demands of the workplace. It can also boost our creativity and problem-solving abilities. For example, if you're having trouble working on a project or studying for an exam or can't seem to solve a problem that is causing you stress, step outside for a breath of fresh air. Take an easy walk outside. You will be surprised by how different that problem seems five, ten or fifteen minutes later.

Studies also show that being in nature has a positive effect on our bodies by reducing cortisol levels, muscle tension, and demands on our cardiovascular systems (it lowers heart rate and blood pressure). Being out in nature often may lead to lower rates of heart disease. The great outdoors can also help you increase your vitamin D level, which is important for your bones, blood cells and immune system. Nature can help decrease your anxiety levels and lessen stress and feelings of anger, frustration and resentment. This is especially true when you add movement and exercise to the equation.

We all know that interacting with nature reduces stress, but it is not clear how long and how often the engagement needs to be, or even what kind of nature experience is best. According to a 2019 study published in *Frontiers in Psychology*, spending just 20 minutes connecting with nature can help lower stress hormone levels. The researchers asked 36 people to spend ten minutes or longer, three days a week, for eight weeks, in an outdoor place where they could interact with nature. Levels of cortisol, a stress hormone, were measured from saliva samples taken before and after nature outings. The people were also instructed not to exercise beforehand and to avoid unrelated stimuli like social media, phone calls, conversations and reading. Spending at least 20 to 30 minutes immersed in a nature setting was associated with the biggest drop in cortisol levels.

After that time, additional stress-reduction benefits accrued more slowly. The time of day and specific settings didn't affect stress levels.

So the next time you need to de-stress or just work on your mental wellbeing, find a nature setting you enjoy and spend some time there. Reduce the distractions and just take it in. Be mindful in that space and you will be enabling nature to help you and your wellbeing.

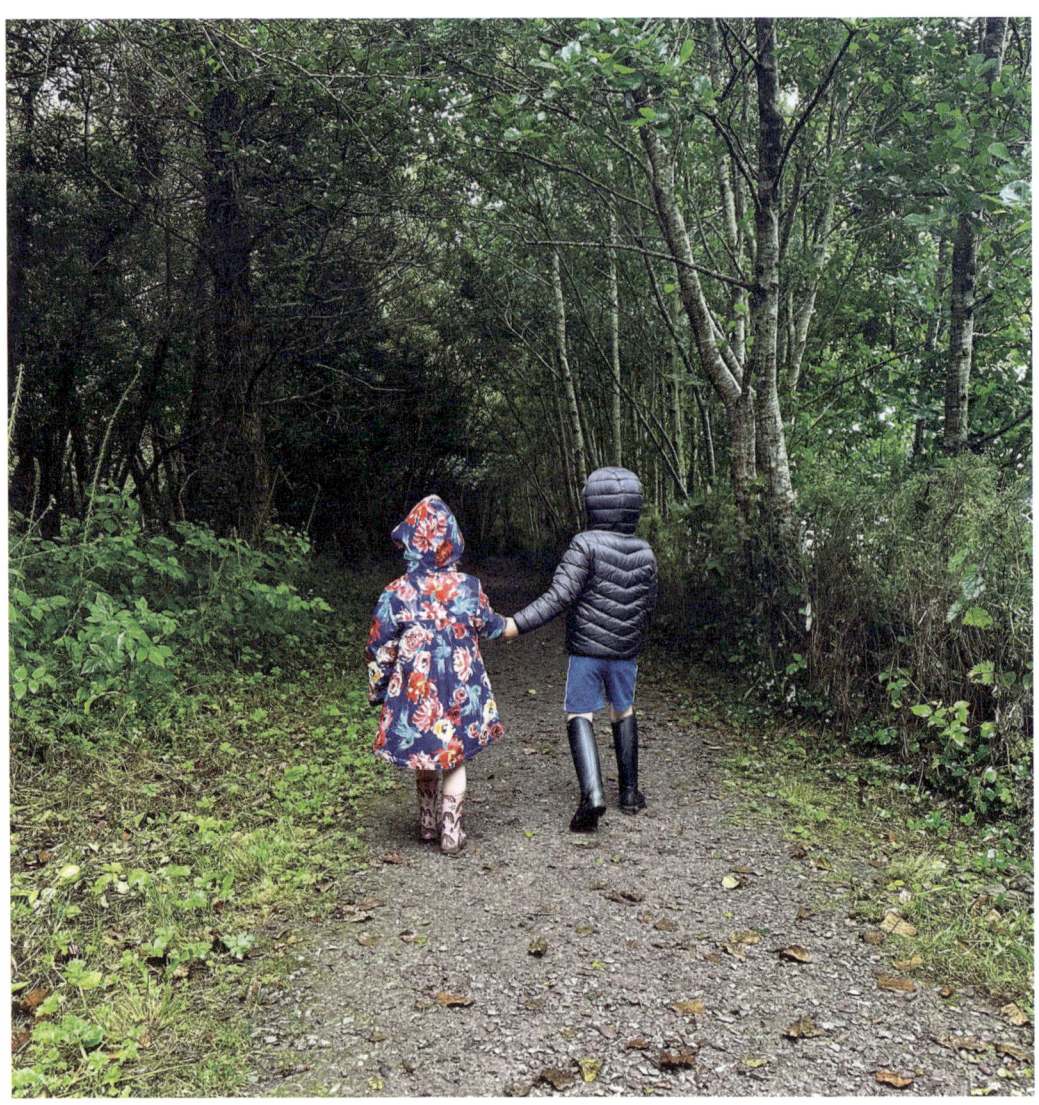

GREEN ZONING

Green zoning means surrounding yourself with trees and plants as much as possible. Doing this on your walk will give you even more benefits.

Peter James, assistant professor in Harvard's T.H. Chan School of Public Health's Department of Environmental Health, said that the effects of trees on us 'translate into long-term changes in the incidence of depression, anxiety, cognitive decline, and chronic diseases including cardiovascular disease and cancer'. That's pretty powerful stuff when you think about just how easy it is to access in your life and your day. On your walk to or from work or even on your lunch break, can you find some trees to be around, to sit beside, to look at, to touch or, if you feel like it, to hug? Find a tree and find better health naturally!

One of the reasons we bought our house is a beautiful tree in the garden. Over the last two years I have spent time clearing around it, I've put a bench beside it and I spend as much time there as I can. There is not a day goes by that I don't get some form of inspiration or release from being near it. When I see it sway and move in the big storms, I find it mesmerising. It is such a symbol of the power of nature and its beauty.

SOME BENEFITS OF WALKING IN FORESTS OR WOODLAND

We have beautiful forests and woodlands to explore in Ireland and walking there is so good for you, your mind and your body. Trees are beautiful, historical and powerful, and they are not only beautiful to look at, they are also cleaning the air around us.

Trees absorb pollutants as well as releasing oxygen, so the air in forests and woodlands is cleaner and better for your health. Just like sea air, air in forests and woodlands is incredible for your body. The seasons bring different smells and colours, meaning no matter when you walk in the woods, two walks will never be the same.

Your lungs will thank you for a woodland walk, as will your cortisol levels. Just being near trees has been shown to reduce the levels of cortisol in our system, which makes us calmer and more relaxed and clears our minds, the better to process life's problems.

Woodlands are known to be restorative environments. The next time you are feeling stressed, try going for a walk in a wood and notice the difference it makes. The clean air, the birdsong, the peacefulness and the light filtering through the trees will all help balance your emotions.

From a physical perspective, woodlands can be great for all your ligaments and tendons too. Paths and trails through woodlands are often uneven, which means that we have to work harder to walk along them, strengthening our muscles and improving our balance in the process. If you have any concerns about your ankles and feet I would recommend wearing a good pair of walking boots with plenty of ankle support, just to be on the safe side.

BLUE ZONING

Blue zoning is exposing yourself to the sea or to water. Water is calming and relaxing and brings with it a lot of health benefits. Proximity to water makes walking even more beneficial, not to mention walking or swimming in it. I think it is one of the many benefits of living in Ireland: we are never too far from water, no matter where we live.

For the past three years I have done long-distance swimming in the sea and in lakes. The power of the sea, the physical and mental effects of it, blow me away. Before and after my swims, I just sit and look at it, tea in hand, decompressing from a hard day. My mood lifts when I just watch the water change patterns, the reflections of nature around it and the sound of it. So much so that I have several saved sea-sound playlists on Spotify that I listen to in the evening. There is something incredibly tranquil about the sound of water and waves.

A study by Carreno et al. looked at the changes in blood pressure, heart rate, sleep quality and mental health of 16 patients after 12 sessions of three different activities (walking by the sea, bathing from the beach and snorkelling). The study found that exposure to blue spaces gave positive results for mental health. Exposure to blue spaces contributes to tension and anger reduction and improves the vigour and mood of oncology patients. In summary, if you are in a bad mood, get out close to water and watch what it will do to your mood and your outlook!

SOME BENEFITS OF WALKING BY THE SEA

We all know that walking by the sea often makes us feel better – the sound of the ocean, the freshness of the sea air, the colours and sounds – but why?

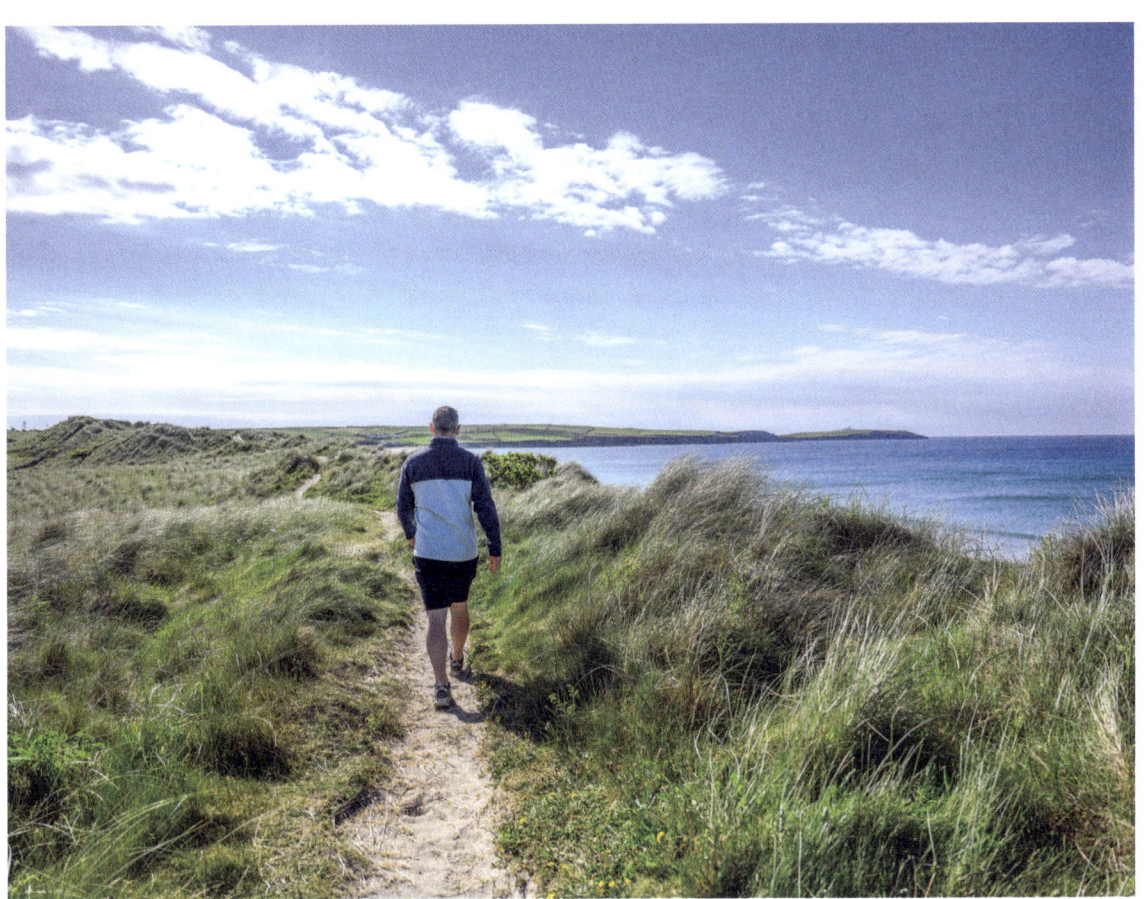

First, it is mindful. You are surrounded by things that will help you to regulate, to slow down, to distract you from the busyness of the world around you. Hearing the sound of the waves, feeling the sand between your toes, tasting the salt in the air will all help you to be in the moment. These are all sensations that help to regulate your emotions and your stress levels and create a sense of calm. It is incredibly powerful.

From a walking perspective, walking on sand is easier on our joints than walking on harder surfaces like pavements and treadmills. Be careful not to walk in very soft or deep sand if you are just starting out as this will really tire out your body and can become a little tricky. The camber of the surface of the beach is really important; a steep beech can put too much pressure on the joints, so be mindful of this. The uneven surface on the beach helps to make muscles stronger as it forces your tendons and ligaments to work a little harder than a flat surface, which can really produce a great workout !

In days gone by people were often sent to the seaside to convalesce, and it turns out that those doctors were on to something: the minerals in the sea air promote respiratory health and have been shown to have other benefits too. Since I moved to west Cork and started spending a lot of time by the sea, I can vouch for just how good I feel for it. Often, the air by the sea is cleaner and fresher, so it's even more beneficial than usual to breathe deeply while you're walking and fill your lungs with the fresh air. It is a great place to try nasal breathing too.

Being by the sea also helps us to connect to nature. We know that nature is one of the superpowers of health, and in this country we are surrounded by some incredible nature. Ireland's coastline has so much amazing wildlife to appreciate, and there's nowhere better to do it than the beach, immersing yourself in all that nature has to offer.

NATURE WALKING IN THE CITY

Sometimes people think you have to be up in the mountains or on a beach or in a forest to get walking in nature. But the reality is you don't. Think about the last time you were in your local town or city. I bet you saw trees, planting and other green things. That is all you need. It is the exposure to these that will deliver the benefits you need. On the way to work tomorrow, choose the green route. Heading to the supermarket tomorrow, park beside the trees or the hedge. Any exposure, however small, will deliver huge benefits, so make those choices and see what happens. Just like taking the opportunities to move that we talked about earlier, opportunities to surround yourself with nature are another thing to choose more often. Seek out greenways, water or any form of nature in your day-to-day life and see what a difference it can make.

HOW TO MAKE YOUR WALK MORE MINDFUL

Mindfulness is one of the buzzwords of the moment. Mindfulness can be pretty much any act of focusing fully on one thing that takes your mind off everything else. Cold-water therapy is a great example of this. It is just so cold that you can't think about anything else and that gives you an incredible sense of wellbeing.

Mindfulness in nature is associated with focusing on what is around you, listening to what is around you and even touching and feeling what is around you. Guided mindfulness is using someone else's voice to help you to focus on the subject and train your mind to be able to do this. Disconnecting from our workday has never been more difficult, and mindfulness teachers have become like personal trainers, helping you to train yourself and your mind to be able to relax more. When combining mindfulness with walking, you not only get the benefits of calmness and relaxation, you also get the physical benefits of the walk itself.

The benefits of mindfulness include:

+ Improved mental health
+ Improved memory
+ Reduced stress
+ Better focus
+ Better sense of control over your life.

BAREFOOT WALKING/GROUNDING

Barefoot walking has become something of a trend in the last few years. It's the closest we get to walking in our most natural state, and I walk barefoot myself as often as possible and anywhere possible. Now, if you have lovely soft feet that are well looked after, walking barefoot may toughen them up a little, especially if you walk outside on the ground. But I like the sensory feedback from walking that way, especially on the grass. Just standing on the grass barefoot, any time of the year, is incredibly empowering and restorative. The beach is another place to connect with the ground and the earth, and walking in the sea barefoot brings those childhood memories flooding back to me. If you struggle to slow your mind down or if you get distracted easily, taking off your shoes and socks can be a great way to create a routine or a process that signals the beginning of a more mindful state for you and your body. In the same way that a warm-up before a run or a class signals the start of that movement, try to make this part of your routine and it will help you hugely to relax and reset.

SOME OF THE BENEFITS OF WALKING BAREFOOT

+ Better control of your foot position when it strikes the ground
+ Improvements in balance, proprioception and body awareness, which can help with pain relief
+ Better foot mechanics, which can lead to improved mechanics of the hips, knees and core
+ Maintaining an appropriate range of motion in your foot and ankle joints as well as adequate strength and stability in your muscles and ligaments
+ Relief from improperly fitting shoes, which may cause bunions, hammer toes or other foot deformities
+ Stronger leg muscles, which support the lower-back region
+ A sense of connection with the ground and the earth
+ A sense of calm.

If you want to walk barefoot, start by walking indoors, build up your distance slowly and rest up if you feel any pain or discomfort. Especially if your feet are soft, ease yourself in. Most of all, enjoy!

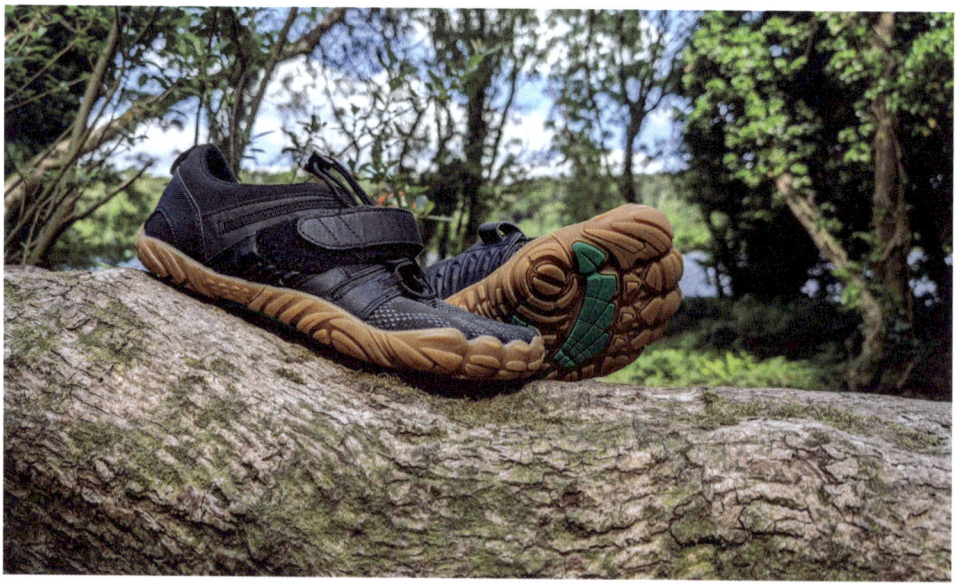

SEASONAL WALKS

WALKING IN WINTER AND AUTUMN

The winter can be a really challenging time to get out and exercise and stay healthy. Here are some simple tips to keep you moving.

Stock up on the base layers

Base layers are one of the key factors in winter walking. They are ultra-warm yet not bulky – tight Lycra-based clothing will warm you up, no matter how cold it is. Several years ago, when we had a spell of heavy snow, I was still training in temperatures of -5°C with just a base layer on, they are that warm. They are meant to be tight-fitting and there are many brands to choose from, such as Under Armour, Canterbury, Columbia and Helly Hansen. They all use different fabrics, so try them on and see which you like best.

Get a good luminous rain jacket

You can be sure it's going to rain when you are planning on going out for a walk, so you need to get a good-quality rain jacket, preferably one that is luminous yellow so you can be seen. Remember, it will get dark early and if you don't ensure you can be seen it makes things very dangerous for you and other road users. I recently bought one by a company called Altura which I find is not only a good rain jacket but also protects against wind chill.

Pick an event

Just like any other time of year, during December and all the winter months you should continue to pick events or classes to go to or have a walking goal to aim for. Beach and mountain walks in winter are epic, blustery and fresh. When I have the right gear on they are probably my favourite types of walk.

Make a list of your goals, which will keep you training and healthy. Have something to train for, something to motivate you to go outside when the couch looks so inviting.

Don't forget gloves and a hat

Most sports shops stock gloves and hats that are specifically made for runners, cyclists and people who do any other type of exercise. If you have a good pair of gloves and a hat you will be far more comfortable when you exercise. If there is a bitter wind you will want to be wrapped up as well as you can, and so much of the heat in your body goes out through your head that a good hat will keep you toasty. I wear woolly hats that my mum knits for some serious warmth, but they can get sweaty. The newer Lycra ones won't as they deal with sweat so well.

Get your friends involved

Sometimes it can be hard to do it alone, so why not enlist your friends or colleagues at work? Why not get a group together once or twice a week to walk? You could have a competition to see who walks the most or adds a new activity to their routine with a small prize at the end of the month – a small incentive just to keep you going. This is something my friends and I do all the time during the year. It makes such a difference!

WALKING IN SPRING AND SUMMER

I always think that spring and summer are energetic months to get outside and walk. As nature awakens and begins to bloom with colour, it is a totally different experience from walking in the other months. Colourful, vibrant, blossoming, reawakening nature is incredible to watch at this time of year. Even the sea looks a different colour on warm sunny days than in the wild winter months.

It is time to lighten the clothing, lengthen the walks and take in the scenery around you. It is also a great time to look at some of the longer and more challenging walks in this book and maybe think of tackling them. Why not use the better weather and longer daylight hours to take your walking to new heights?

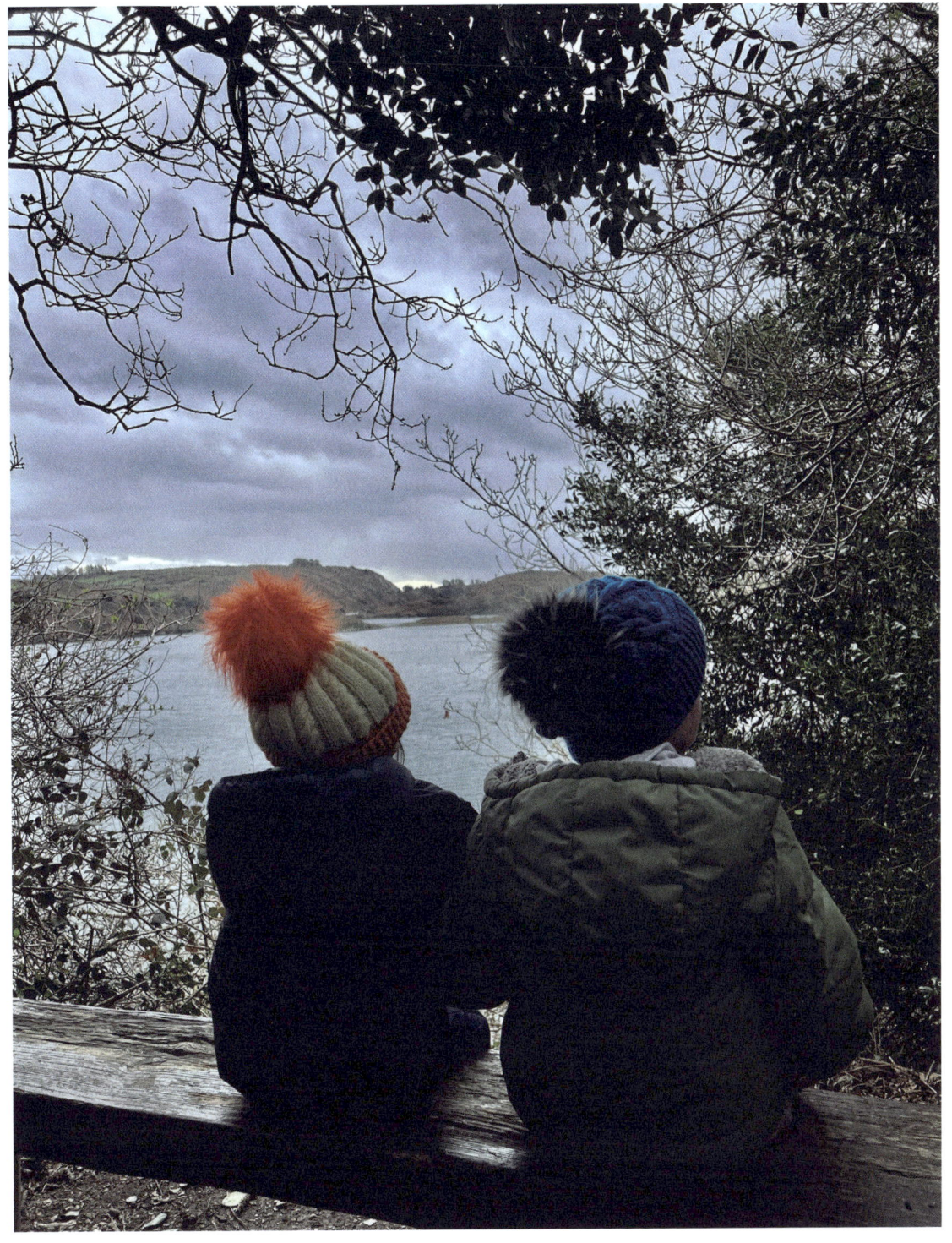

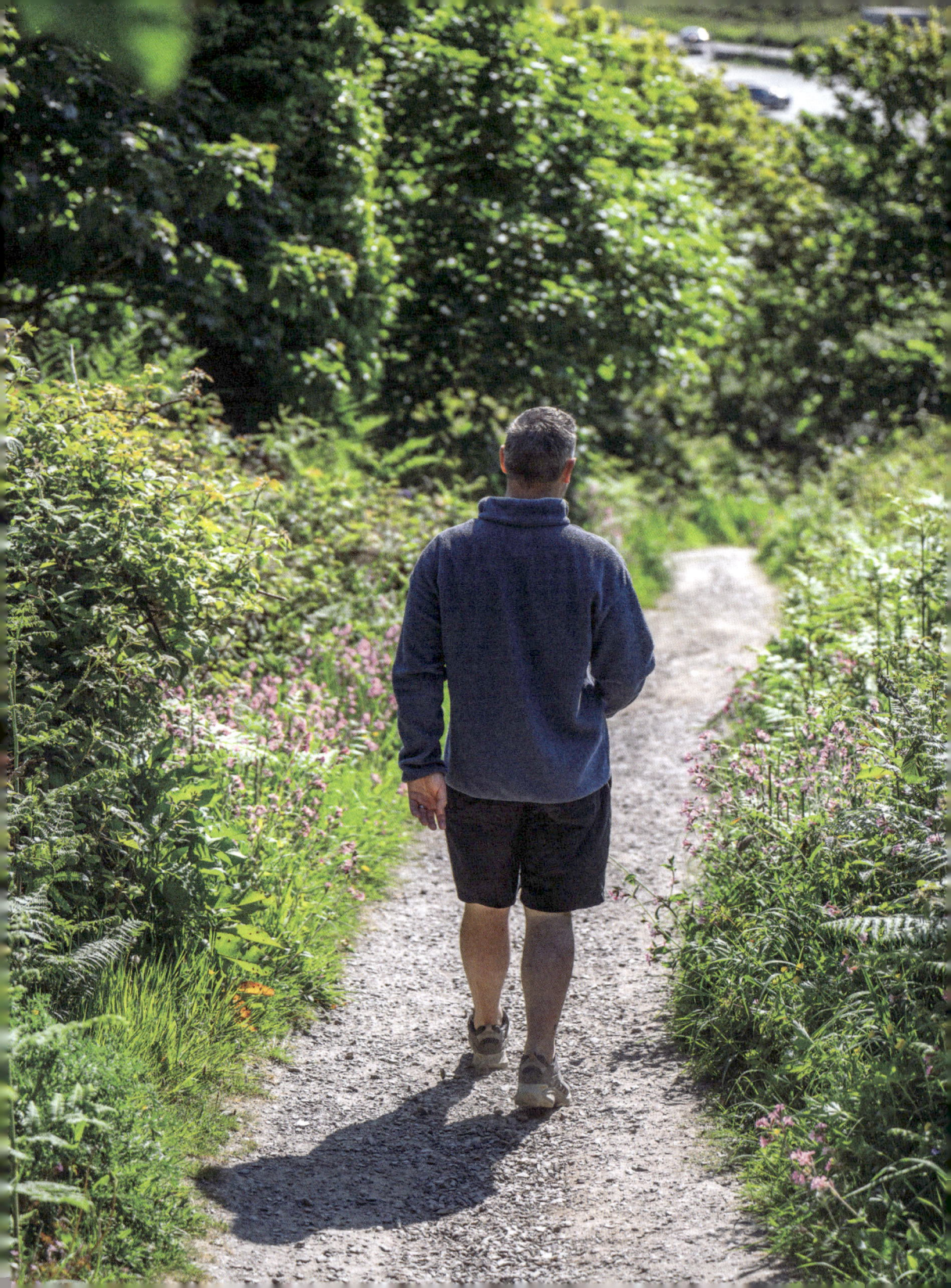

CHAPTER FIVE

SOME OF MY FAVOURITE WALKS IN IRELAND

We live in an incredible country for walking and so many people don't realise just what is on their doorstep. Here I want to give you some of my favourite walks in each province. They are suitable for different levels of fitness and ability. You'll see that the highest peak in each province features on the list. I have been lucky enough to climb them several times with the Four Peaks Challenges that I take some of my corporate wellness groups on. They are epic, beautiful climbs but also tough; you should ideally tackle them with a guide and a group of other keen hillwalkers. Why not set climbing one of them as your goal as you get fitter and stronger?

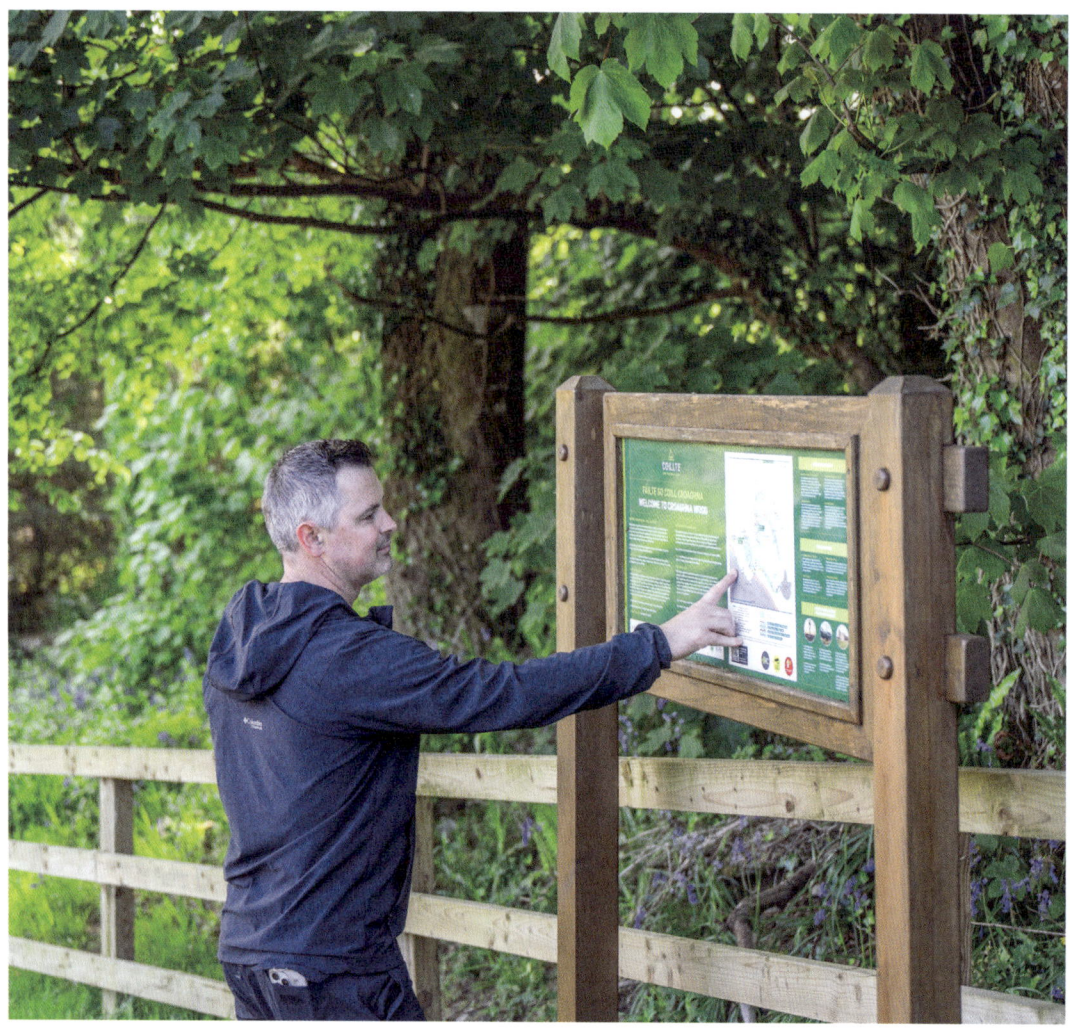

STAYING SAFE

Safety is so important when out walking, especially as you begin to take on some longer and more challenging hikes. Here are some really simple tips to keep you safe when out for a walk. Some may seem obvious, but you can never be too careful.

PLAN YOUR ROUTE

When planning your route, it is important to be realistic about your fitness levels and make sure you have the fitness to tackle the route you are thinking of doing. Chose a trail that is well marked – this is something that Ireland has really got better at over the last ten years or so. Loop walks are a good choice as you don't have to double back over the same track and each step is taking you closer to home. Even if you are walking with a group, take a look at a map before you set off so that you have an idea of the route in your mind. It is also nice to know a little bit more about where you are going and the scenery you are going to see. A little bit of background information can make the whole experience so much more enjoyable, something that we see with our walking groups, especially on our Camino walking trips.

TELL SOMEONE

If you have planned your route and checked the map, you will know roughly what time you'll be back at the car. It is always a good idea to tell a friend where you're going and what time you'll be finished. Then text them when you get back to your car.

BREAK IN YOUR SHOES

When people get enthusiastic about walking, they always buy shiny new boots. Every single group we work with does this, no matter how many times we advise against it. After all, who doesn't love new things? But be careful. You don't want to undo all your preparation by wearing your boots for the first time on the hills or when out for your walks. That is a recipe for disaster and I can guarantee you that you will be getting plenty of blisters along the way if you do. No matter what socks you have bought, your shiny new boots need to be broken in and given time to settle in. Be kind to your feet: wear your hiking boots around the house and on short walks out and about, or even to work if you can. Do this for a few weeks and then wear them on a shorter walk or trek and see how you get on. Blisters can make a walk so uncomfortable so let's try to avoid them as best we can.

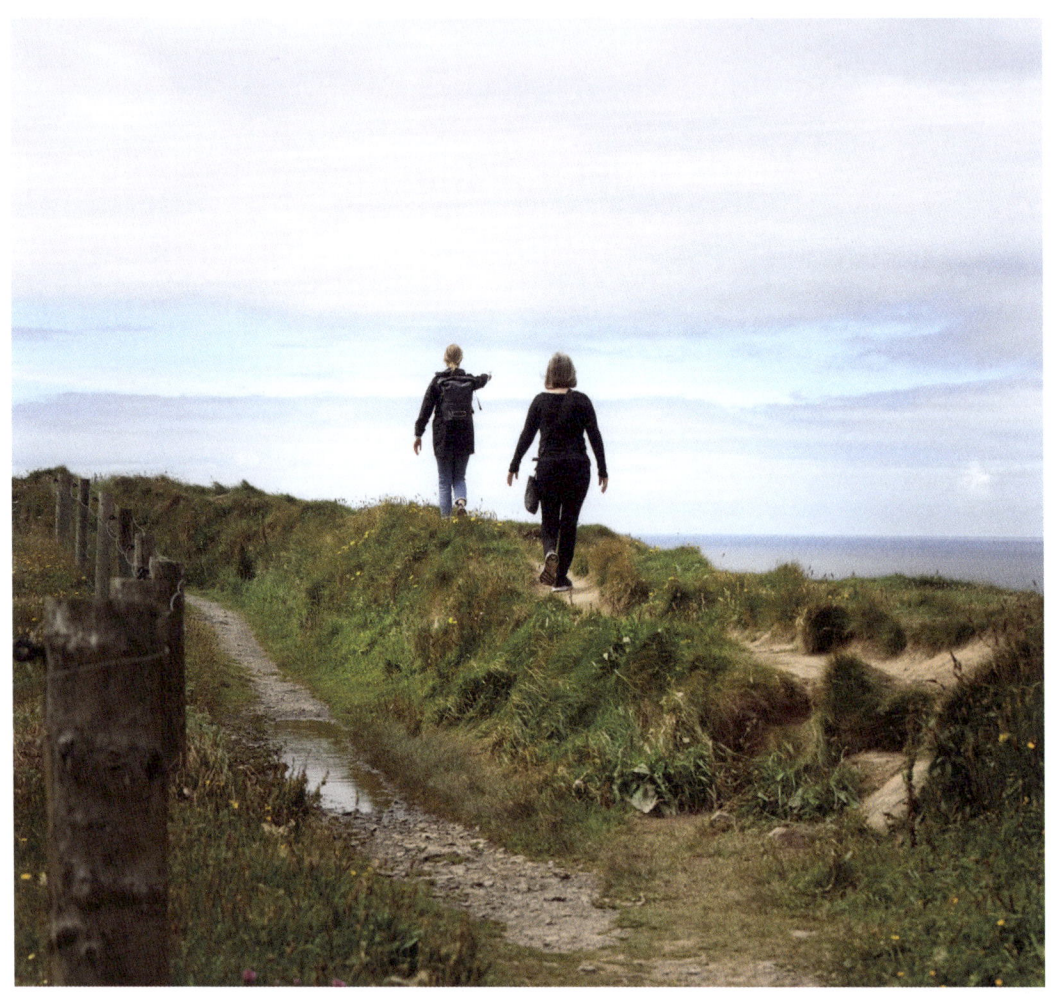

START EARLY IN THE DAY

Not only is it cooler earlier in the day, it makes the whole walk more enjoyable by giving you more time to stop for breaks, take photos and admire the landscape around you. We sometimes tend to rush our walks, but learning to take more time to appreciate what's around you will give you so much more benefit from the walk. And there is something magical about being out in nature early in the morning, especially in the summer months.

BRING SNACKS AND WATER

There are plenty of recipes for snacks in this book that you could bring with you; or you can buy/make your own. But snacks and water are essential, and the longer the hike or the walk, the more you need to bring.

BE PREPARED FOR BAD WEATHER

The weather can change so quickly, especially as you start going higher. Even if you are kitted out properly, if the weather turns and you have even the slightest concern, don't be afraid to call it quits and turn back. Safety always comes first.

EMERGENCIES

Prevention is always key. By knowing the weather and planning out a route, and having a map or guide, you are giving yourself the best chance of a great walk. But if the worst happens and you are injured, lost or need help, Mountain Rescue can be reached by calling 112 or 999.

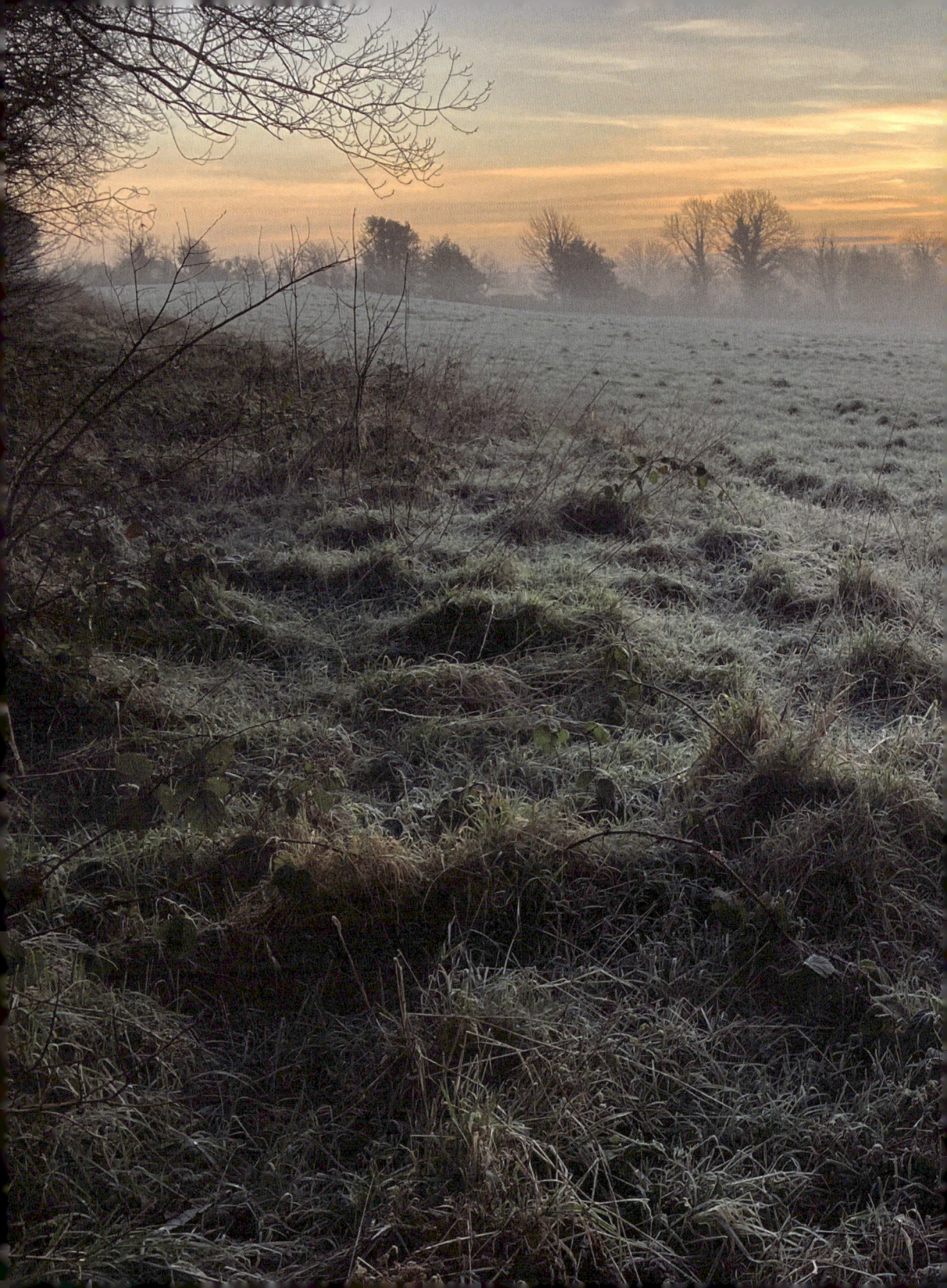

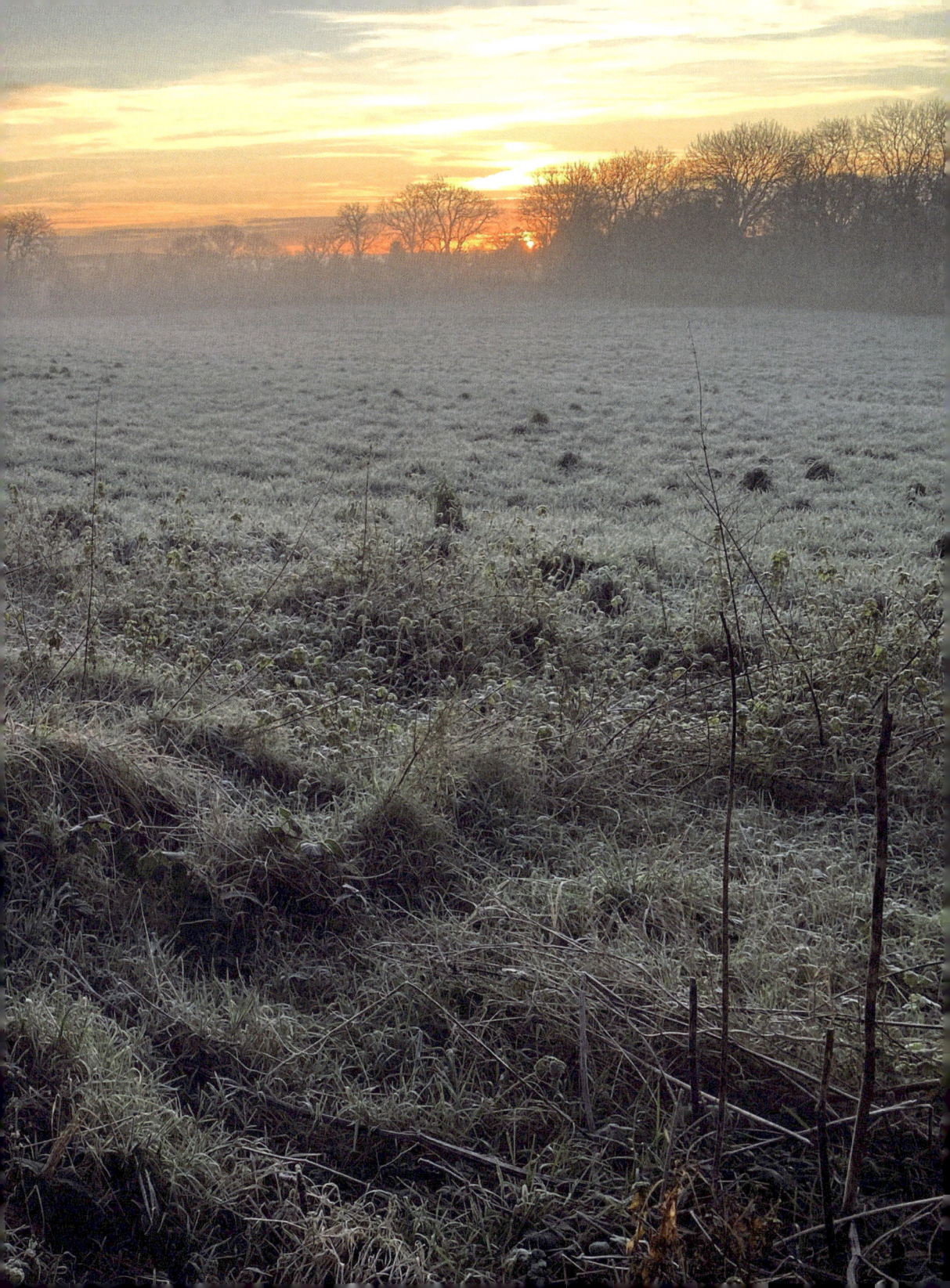

LEINSTER

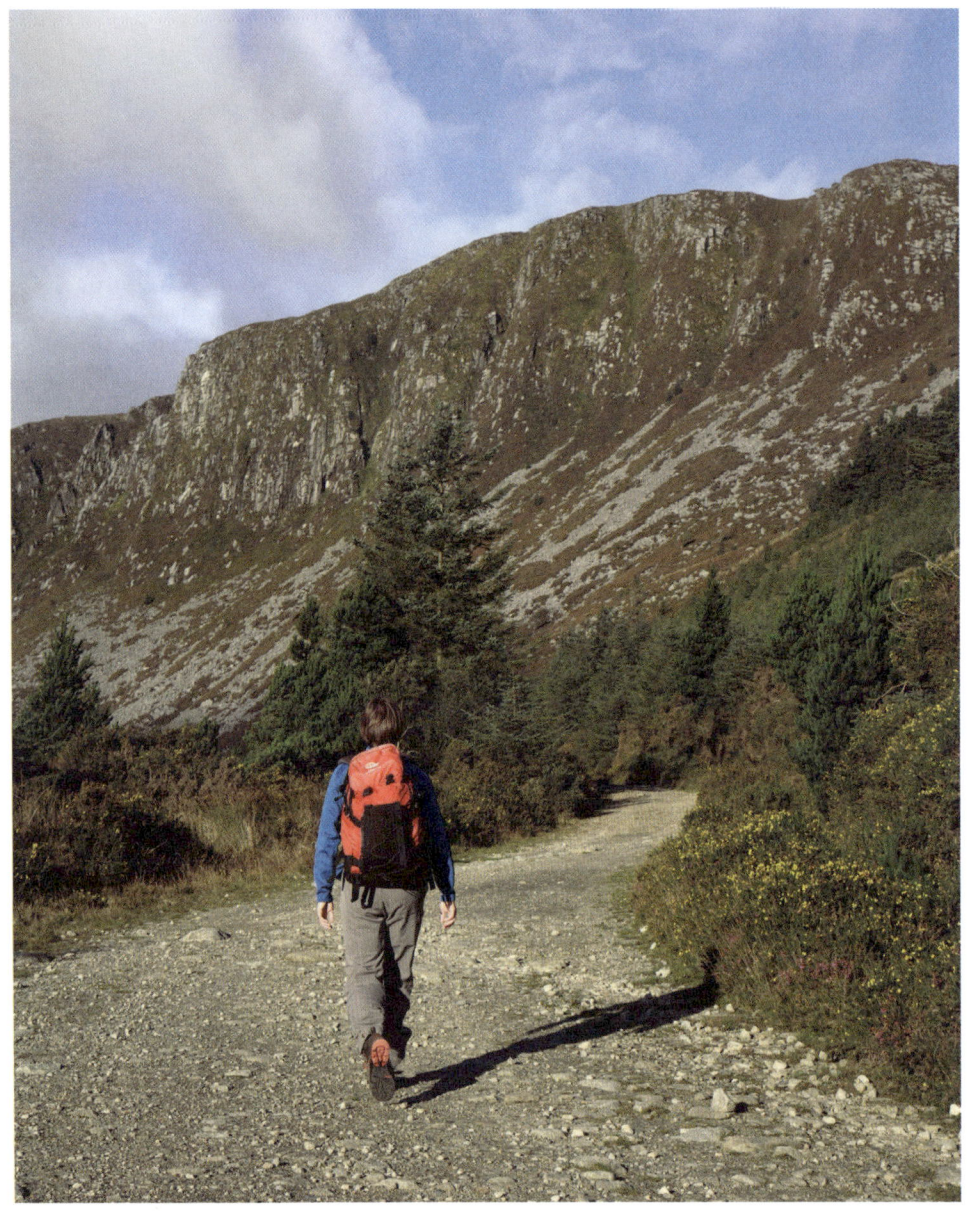

LUG NA COILLE, CO. WICKLOW

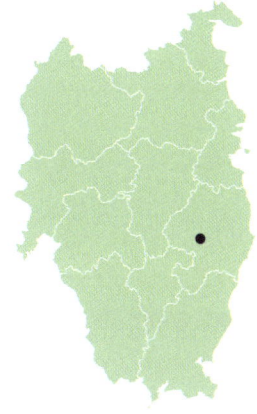

DISTANCE: 10–16KM

DIFFICULTY: HARD

TIME: 5–8 HOURS

This is one of my favourite climbs in Ireland, but the weather can change really quickly, so it is a route to be taken with some caution. There are a few different routes, but my own favourite is via Fraughan Rock Glen, which offers a more gradual, gentle and scenic route to the summit, at 925 metres. This is the highest point in Leinster and in good weather there are superb views across the Wicklow Mountains, Mount Leinster and even across the Irish Sea to Wales!

The route starts at the site of the memorial stone to the 1798 rebellion and travels up a forest road into Fraughan Rock Glen. From here the route gains elevation and eventually you will reach the broad northern ridge of the mountain. Then head for the summit cairn, where you can place your own rock to mark your achievement.

From the summit, head east, down another broad ridge, taking in the superb views – on a clear day – before dropping down to Art's Lough and into the forest. Keep going and you will reach a forest track and the final leg down through the trees and back to your starting point.

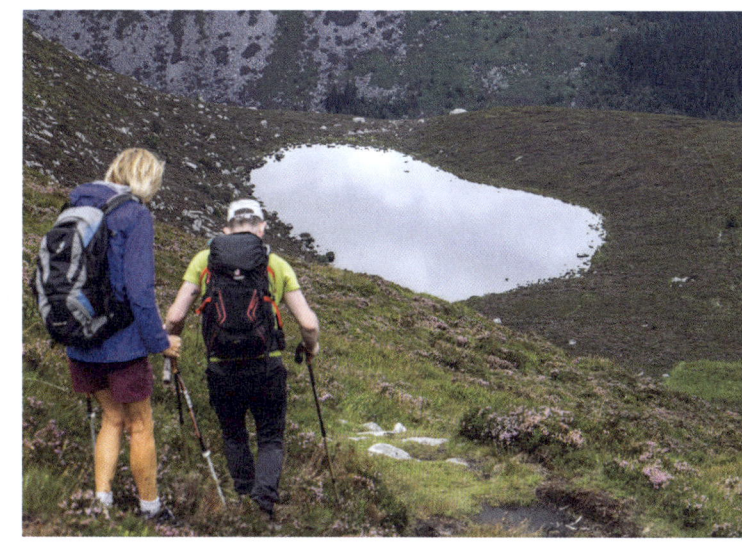

DJOUCE, CO. WICKLOW

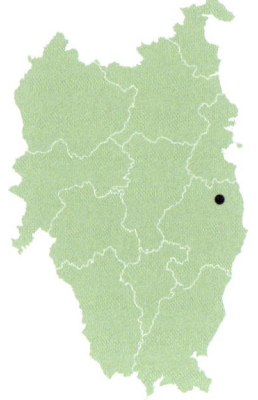

DISTANCE: 14KM

DIFFICULTY: EASY TO MODERATE

TIME: 1.5–4 HOURS

This hike has a special place in my heart. When I was in first year in college, a family friend took me here and it was one of those moments that really kick-started my whole journey into fitness and endurance events. I struggled on that day but went back each Sunday until it got easier, and eventually started running it.

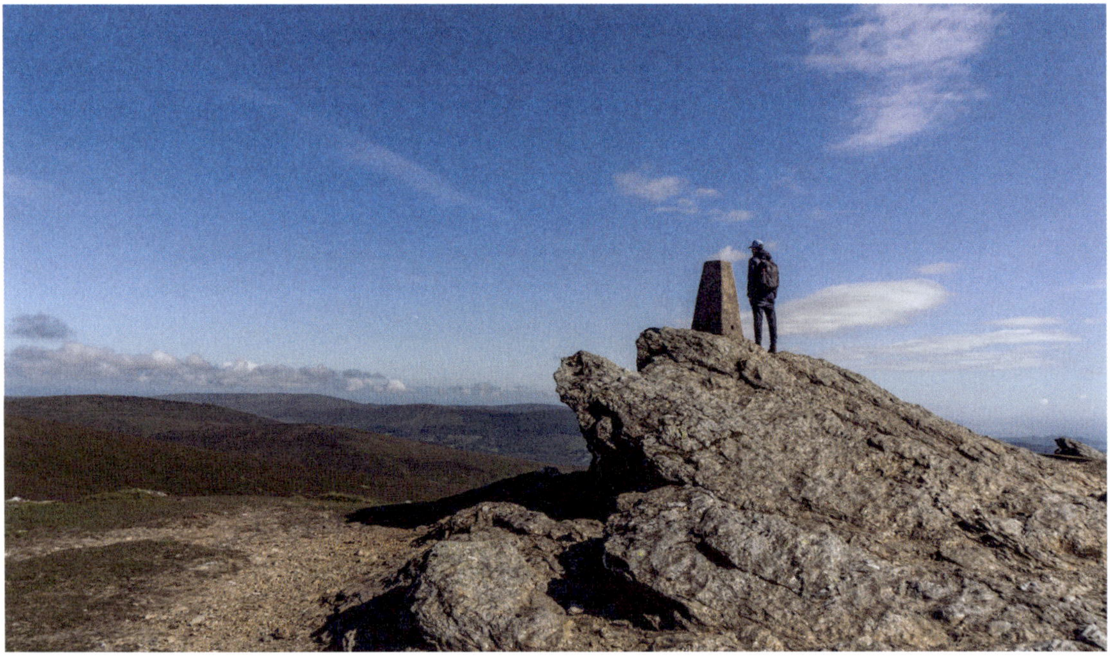

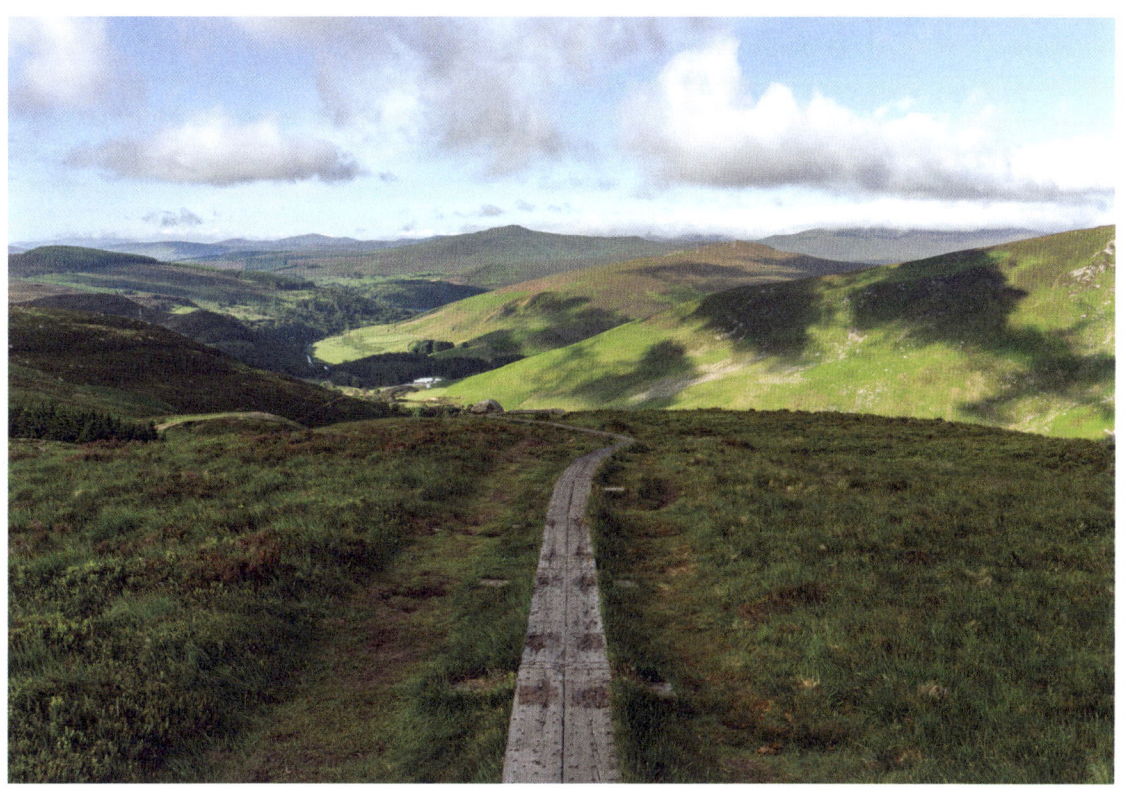

Djouce once formed part of the Powerscourt Estate, a property with numerous roads and drives back in the day, including Lady's Drive and Earl's Drive, that now form part of the forest trail and road network.

Views from Djouce include the Dargle River valley and Powerscourt Waterfall, the highest waterfall in Ireland and Britain. Djouce Mountain (725m) lies to the south west in the Wicklow Mountains National Park, and it is along the Wicklow Way.

There are two walking trails to explore at Djouce. The Blue Loop (4.5km, 1.5 hours, easy) follows one of the old driving roads where you get occasional views over to the deer park and the Powerscourt Waterfall. The Deerpark loop (9km, 3 hours, moderate) takes in the Paddock Ponds, which were a water source for the renowned Powerscourt fountains. It also gives you panoramic views over the Sugarloaf, Bray, Killiney Hill and Dublin Bay to Howth and along the Wicklow Mountains. The routes from the car park are trail marked with signposts, and it's a really great place for families too.

MAULIN, CO. WICKLOW

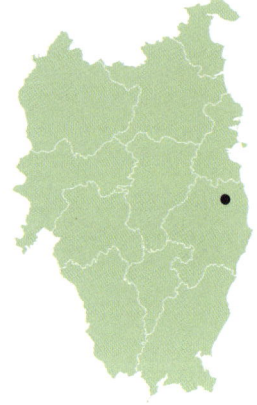

DISTANCE: 7KM

DIFFICULTY: MODERATE

TIME: 2–3 HOURS

This walk is across the valley from Djouce Mountain and starts at Crone Woods, another access point for climbing to the summit of Djouce. The Maulin Mountain Loop brings you high up on to the summit slopes of Maulin Mountain, with trail markers guiding you all the way to the top and all the way back down. It's a brilliant route that follows a fairly gentle climb through the forest, where you can appreciate a beautiful variety of tree species, such as Douglas fir, larch, Corsican pine, Sitka spruce and Scots pine.

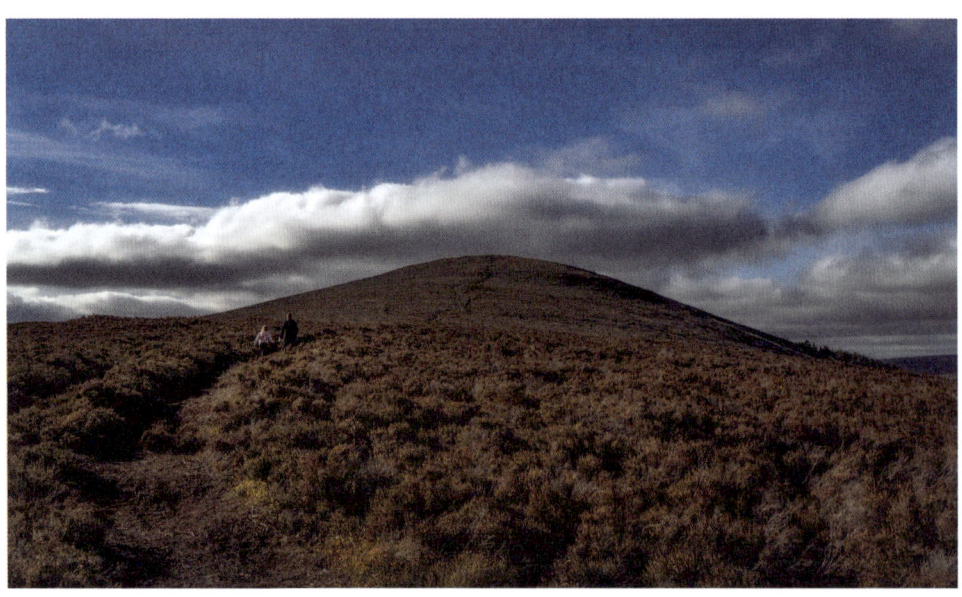

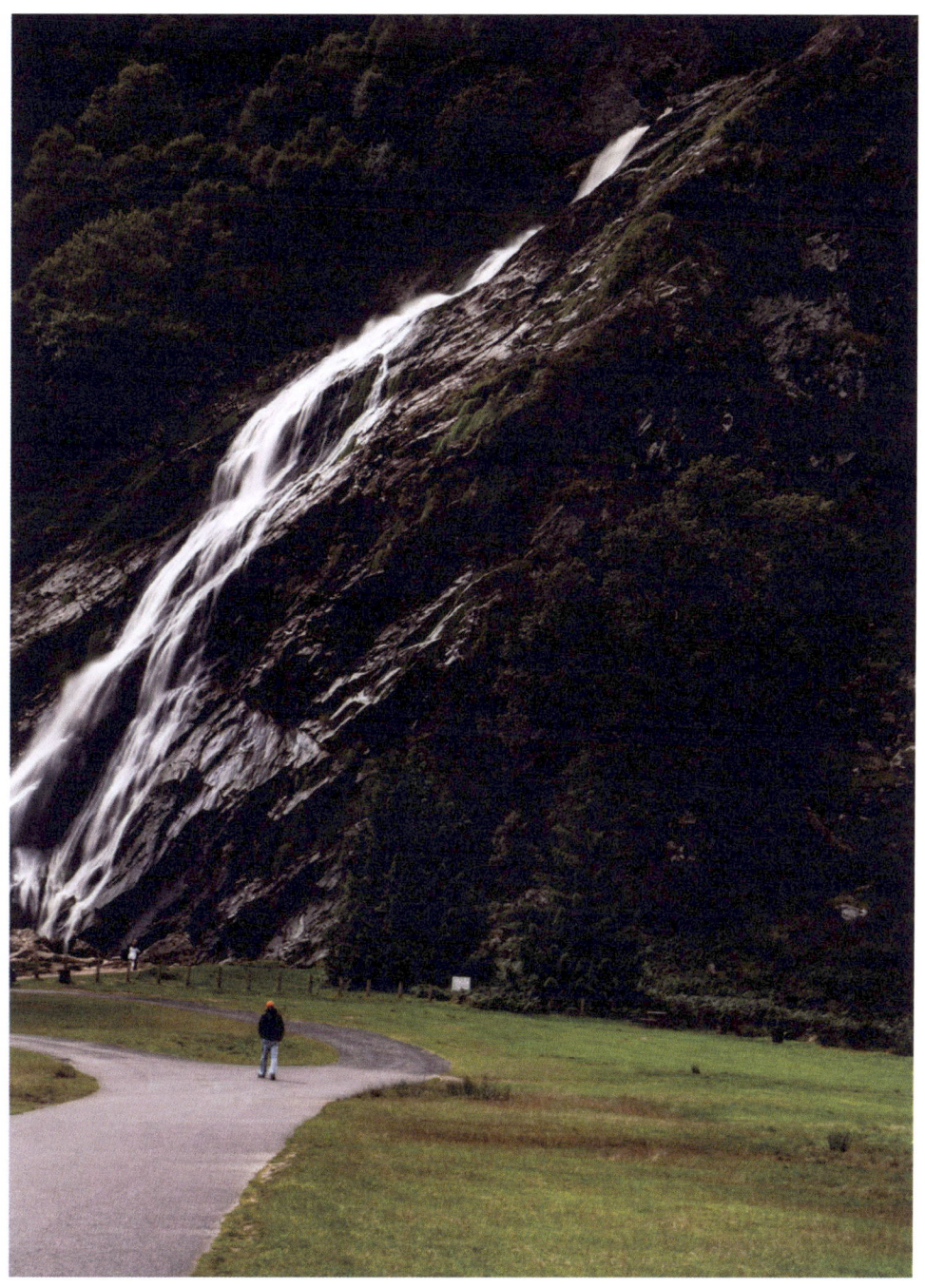

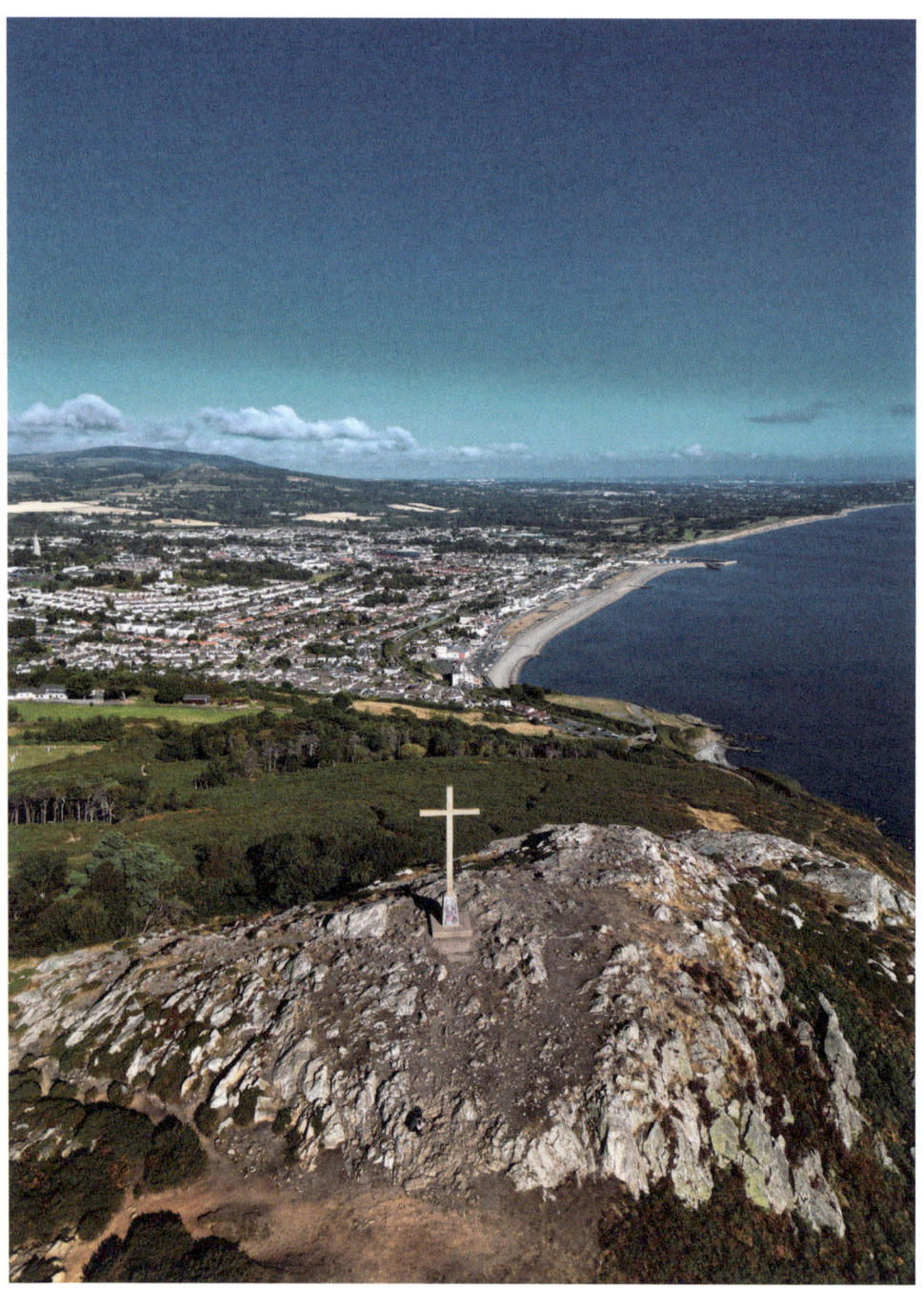

BRAY HEAD, CO. WICKLOW

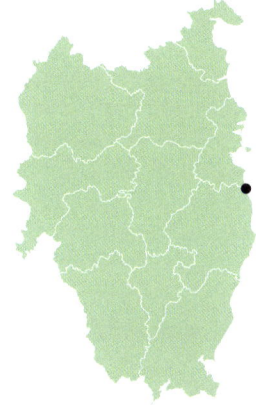

DISTANCE: 9.8KM

DIFFICULTY: EASY

TIME: 90 MINUTES

Bray Head Walk is a 9.8-kilometre loop trail where you can get some really beautiful scenic views of County Dublin and Bray itself. It can be chilly on a windy day, so wrap up!

While this walk isn't overly difficult and can be enjoyed by the entire family, be prepared for tough patches and a little scrambling. The hard work will be worth it once you reach the iconic stone cross that sits atop the hill and take in the incredible views of Bray and Dublin Bay.

You can follow the trail the whole way to the top of the hill but be careful when walking in adverse weather conditions as part of the trail is a tree-lined, dirt path that can get mucky – best to leave your good shoes at home! The stone cross found at the end of the walk was erected there in 1950 to mark the Holy Year.

On your way down just follow the same path or – if you want to take the scenic route – you can follow the path to the south. This path veers off to the right, coming out on the Bray–Greystones road at Windgates. Follow the path back to Bray, passing the golf club; keep straight until you reach Newcourt Road, then make a right turn and follow the road to the end.

Turn right to finish at the seafront, where you can reward your efforts with an ice cream or hot drink.

HILL OF HOWTH, CO. DUBLIN

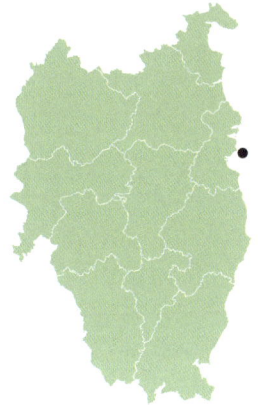

DISTANCE: 6KM

DIFFICULTY: EASY TO MODERATE

TIME: 90 MINS

Another walk that was a weekly staple when I lived in Dublin and became one of my regular training runs for my marathon and Ironman training, the Hill of Howth is hard to beat for all levels of fitness. Setting off from the fishing village of Howth, you have several different options and can make the walk as long or as short as you want. The trails are marked with a map and signposts.

The trail leads you along the charming harbour before climbing away from the village around Howth Cliff and on to the breathtaking clifftops. The terrain may be rough in parts, so walking boots are recommended. Taking the 7.8km clifftop loop gives you incredible views of Dublin's most spectacular coastline, islands and Howth Harbour Lighthouse as you climb to the car park at the top of the hill and back down. Keep an eye on the sea for seals and a whole host of wildlife along the way, as well as the ships coming into the port. I am always astonished that this walk is so close to the city.

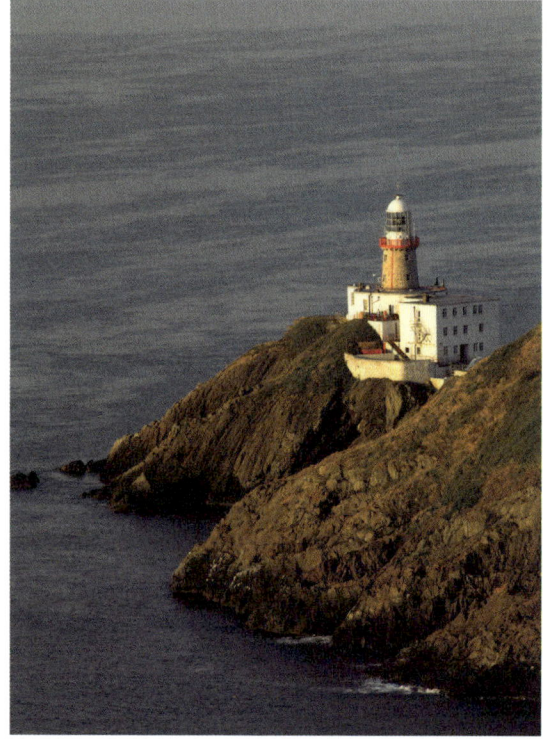

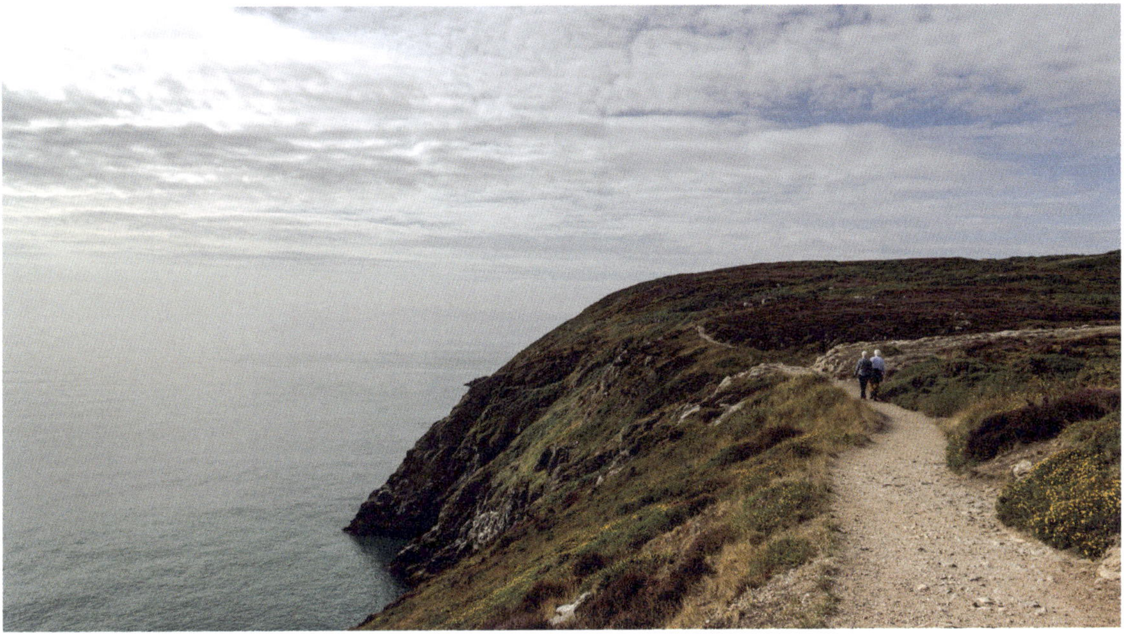

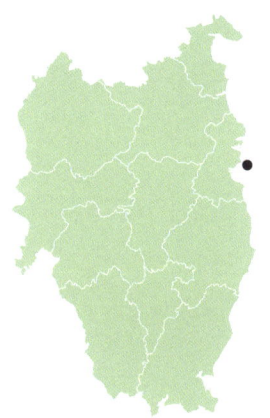

HOWTH CLIFF PATH, CO. DUBLIN

DISTANCE: 6KM

DIFFICULTY: EASY

DURATION: 2 HOURS

Pack a sandwich, pull on your hiking boots and jump on the Dart in Dublin city centre, and just 30 minutes later you'll be in the fishing village of Howth. With a history that can be traced back to the Vikings, this lively little spot is known for its friendly harbour seals, seafood restaurants and breathtaking natural scenery. It's also home to one of the best coastal walks around: the Howth Cliff Path. Running to around 6km, the trail starts at the Dart station before hitting some of the most exhilarating coastal scenery around. Expect sheer drops, jagged cliff-edges, heather-filled hills, boggy fields and a truly beautiful lighthouse perched at the end of the peninsula.

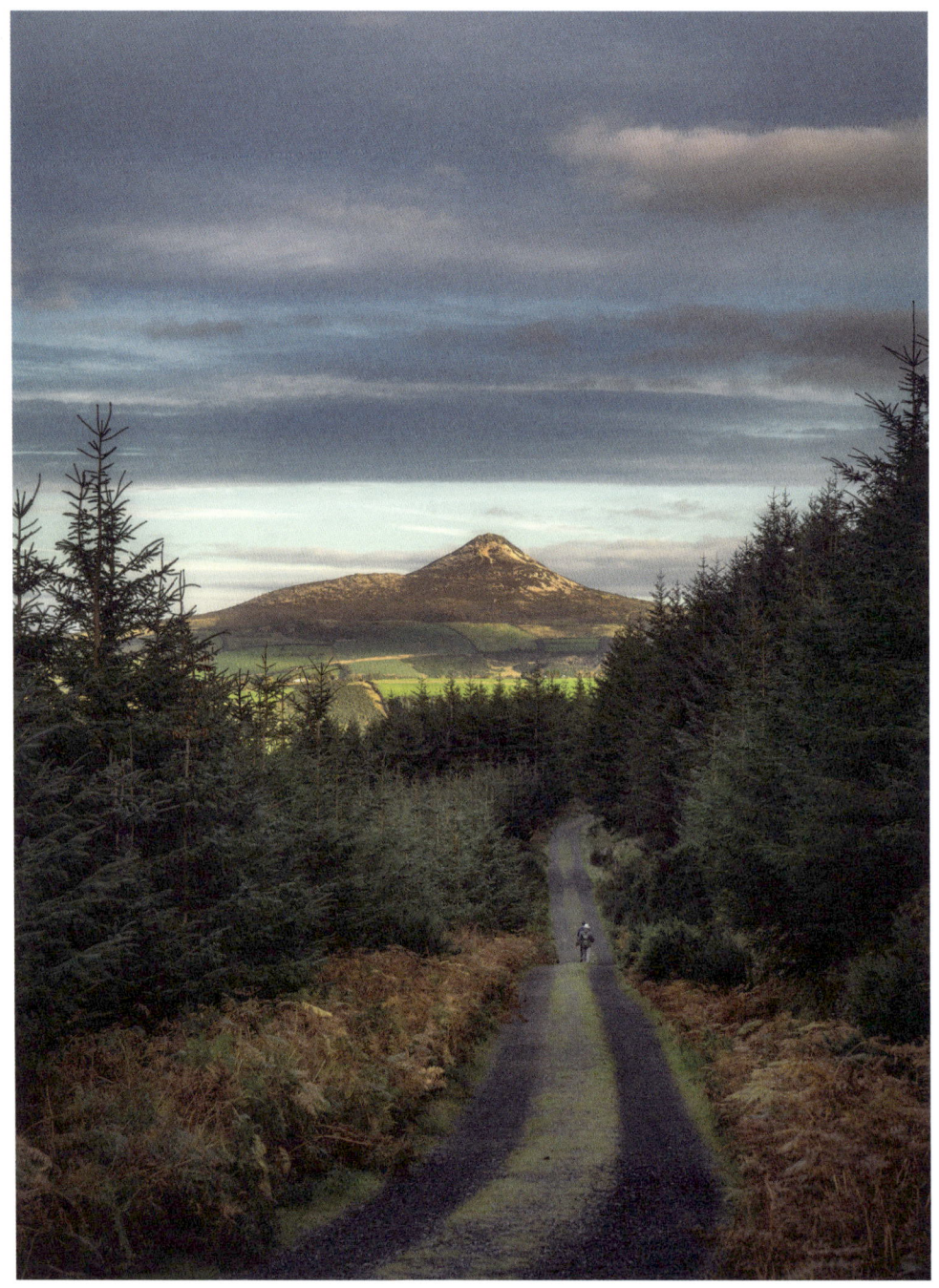

THE SUGAR LOAF, CO. WICKLOW

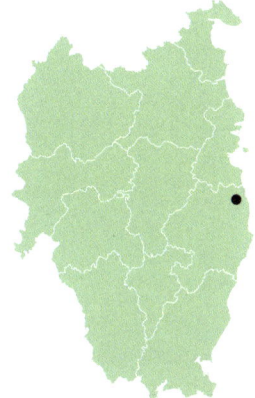

DISTANCE: 8–9KM

DIFFICULTY: MODERATE

TIME: 1–2 HOURS

The Great Sugar Loaf Mountain dominates the skyline as you drive south from Dublin into Wicklow and it's a mountain that lots of us know and remember from our childhoods. It is a challenging family hike and a great one to add to your bucket list.

The short walk from the car park on Red Lane follows a path that meanders left and then right towards the summit. The last thirty metres or so are the hardest, but the views make it all worthwhile.

The longer walk starts at the GAA club, where you will see the trail markers. Follow the path, which will eventually swing left towards the summit.

If you feel like a treat afterwards you can head to Avoca or Enniskerry for a revitalising lunch!

MUNSTER

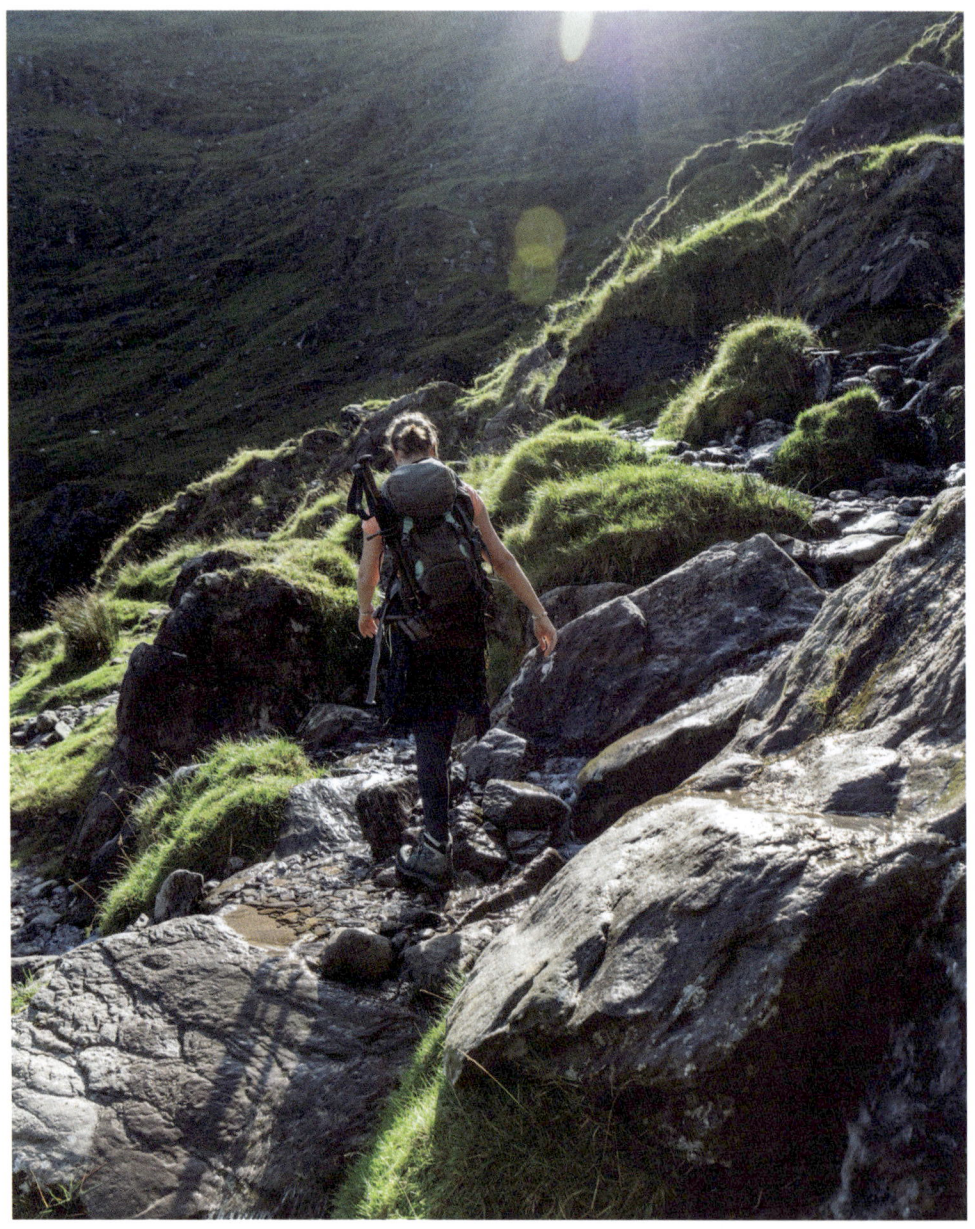

CARRAUNTOOHIL, CO. KERRY

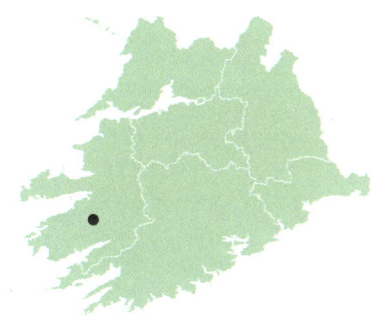

DISTANCE 11–12KM

DIFFICULTY: HARD

TIME: 5–7 HOURS

I have climbed Carrauntoohil several times with corporate groups and, as Ireland's tallest peak, there is something epic about it, especially on a clear day when you stand at the cross at the top looking at the scenery around you.

The easiest place to start is at Cronin's Yard. There are a car park, coffee shop and toilets here, which make it an ideal place to start and finish. This is a serious hike, like any of the four tallest peaks, and not one to be undertaken unless you are sure you are ready for it. It is a great route to do with a guide as you get to learn so much about the area along the way.

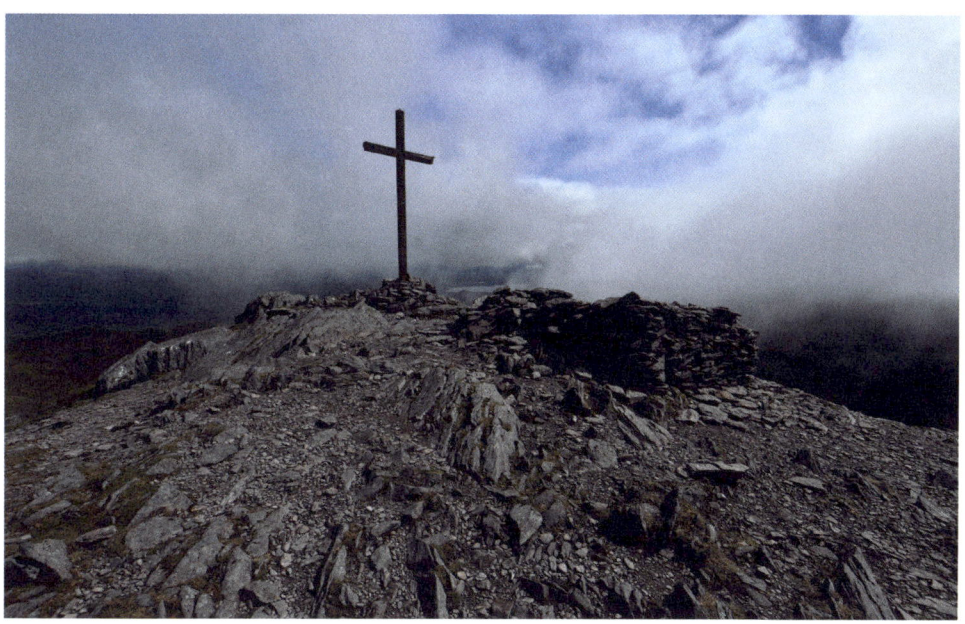

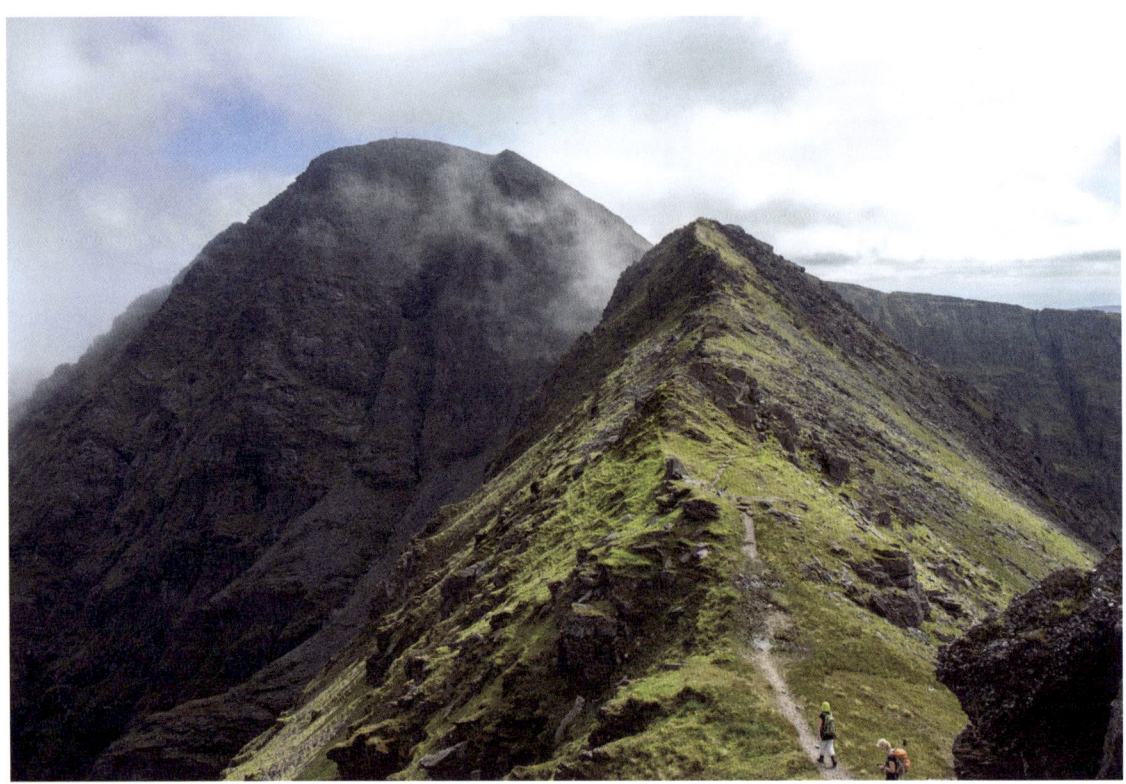

From the start at Cronin's Yard, follow the path until you meet the main Hag's Glen track shortly after the Gaddagh River crossing. Turning left, continue into the Hag's Glen, passing between loughs Gouragh and Callee. After ascending a short rise the path becomes less distinct as it crosses an area of waterlogged ground before arriving at the foot of the Devil's Ladder. The Devil's Ladder itself is a steep gully filled with loose scree and boulders. It is now quite unstable in places as so many people are climbing the mountain, so care should be taken, particularly when it is icy or in wet weather. If it is busy when you are climbing, make sure you leave space between you and the people in front of you as they can dislodge rocks and other debris that could fall towards you.

At the top of the Devil's Ladder, bear right and onto the long summit slope of the mountain. The track is initially hard to make out, but it becomes more obvious as you gain height. You will notice that it seems to branch off in several places, but they all lead to the cross at the top. There is also a very handy wind shelter at the top, should you need it to have some food. Return via the same route or the Brother O'Shea's Gully route, both of which will bring you back to Cronin's Yard.

LOOP HEAD CLIFF WALK, CO. CLARE

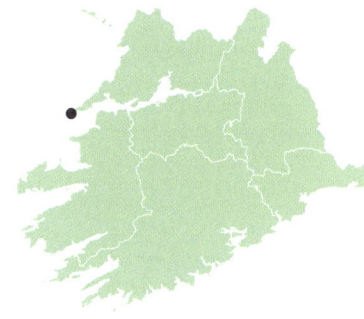

DISTANCE: 1.5KM

DIFFICULTY: EASY

TIME: 1–2 HOURS

The Loop Head Cliff Walk is a really easy one- to two-hour loop walk from the lighthouse car park and around the spectacular headland on Ireland's wild Atlantic coast. Great for families and scenery, the Loop Head peninsula is steeped in history and folklore, and is known as one of the Wild Atlantic Way's most dramatic headlands. It's a great place to birdwatch and to spot dolphins.

Park at the lighthouse car park and the loop will bring you right back around to the car park at the end of your walk.

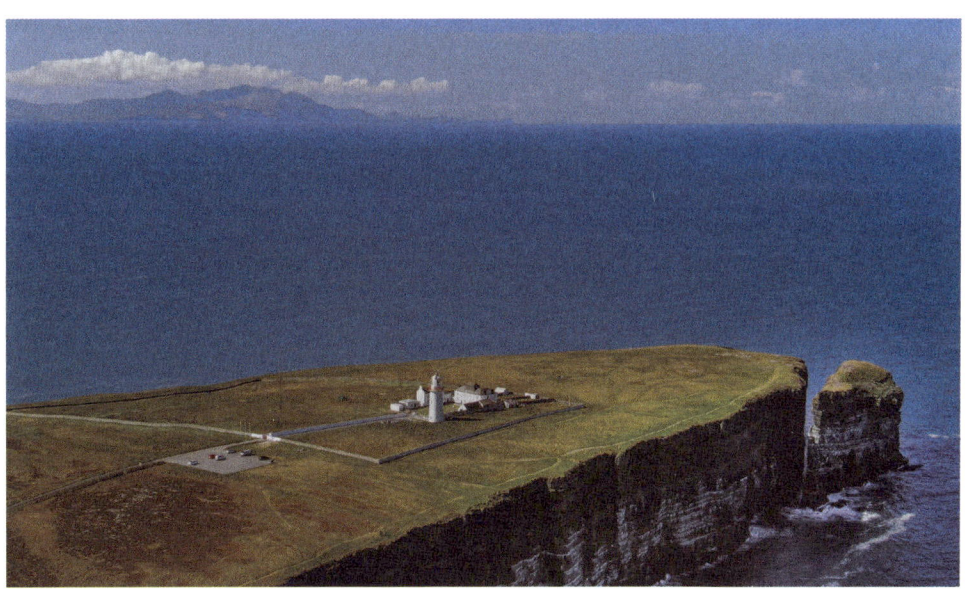

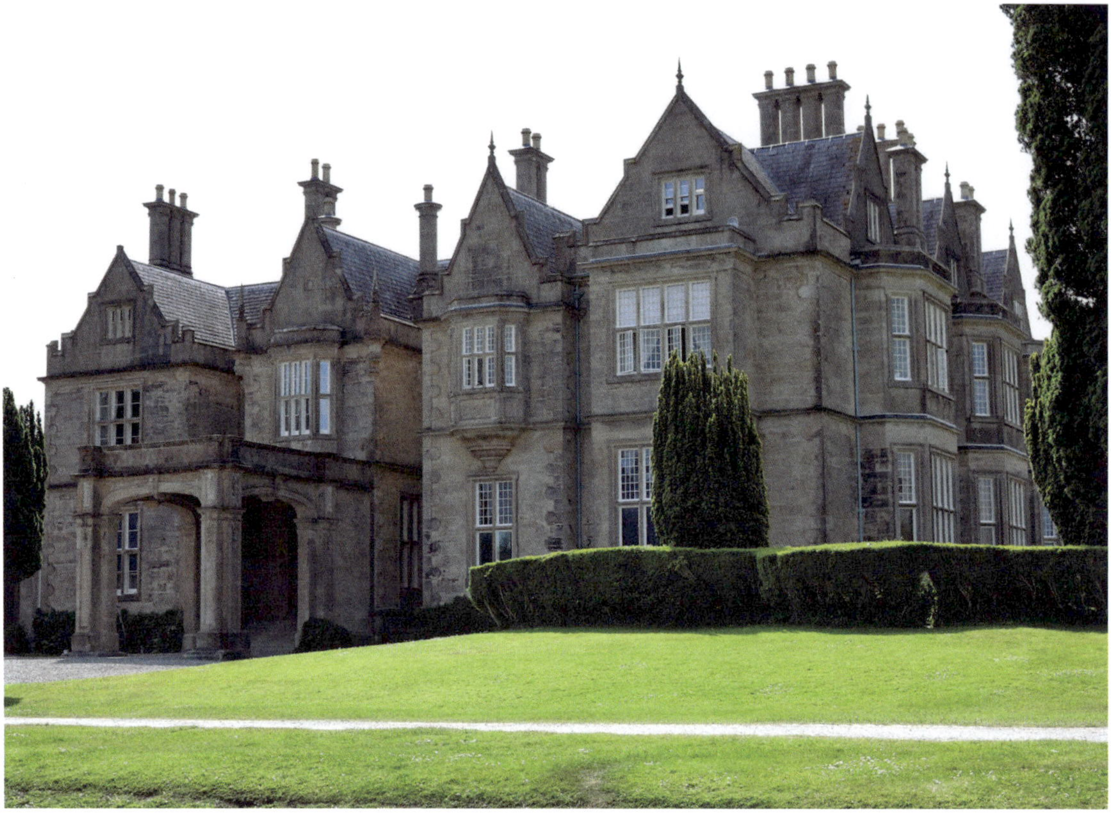

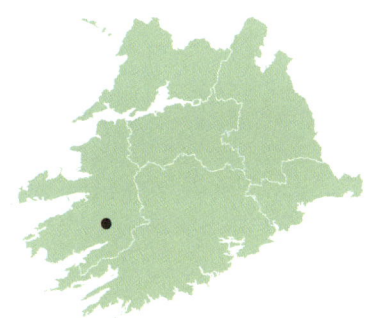

MUCKROSS LAKE LOOP, CO. KERRY

DISTANCE: 15KM

DIFFICULTY: EASY

TIME: 3.5 HOURS

Muckross House, and the Muckross Estate, is a walkers' paradise. It's close to Killarney town, with amazing scenery and walks to suit every single fitness and ability level. You have so many to choose from, but here is just one of the longer ones.

Park in Muckross House car park, a great base to start and finish, with a great restaurant for some food afterwards. Start the walk by making your way along the signposted route from the nineteenth-century Muckross House. Quiet paths take you away from the estate and down to the small beaches and rocky coves of Muckross Lake with views across the lake, bringing you to the Muckross Penisula and Reenadinna Woods. You can stop for refreshments at Dinis Cottage – which has operated as a tea room for more than 200 years – before going behind the cottage to join a short path that leads to the Meeting of the Waters, where Killarney's Upper Lake flows down to join the lower loughs. Tracks by the lake and wooded paths will lead you back to Muckross House and the car park.

Not long before you reach the house, if you'd like to make the walk more challenging, you can take a detour to the top of Torc Waterfall. It's a short but really lovely hike to the top of the waterfall – you could also tackle this circuit on its own, if you'd prefer.

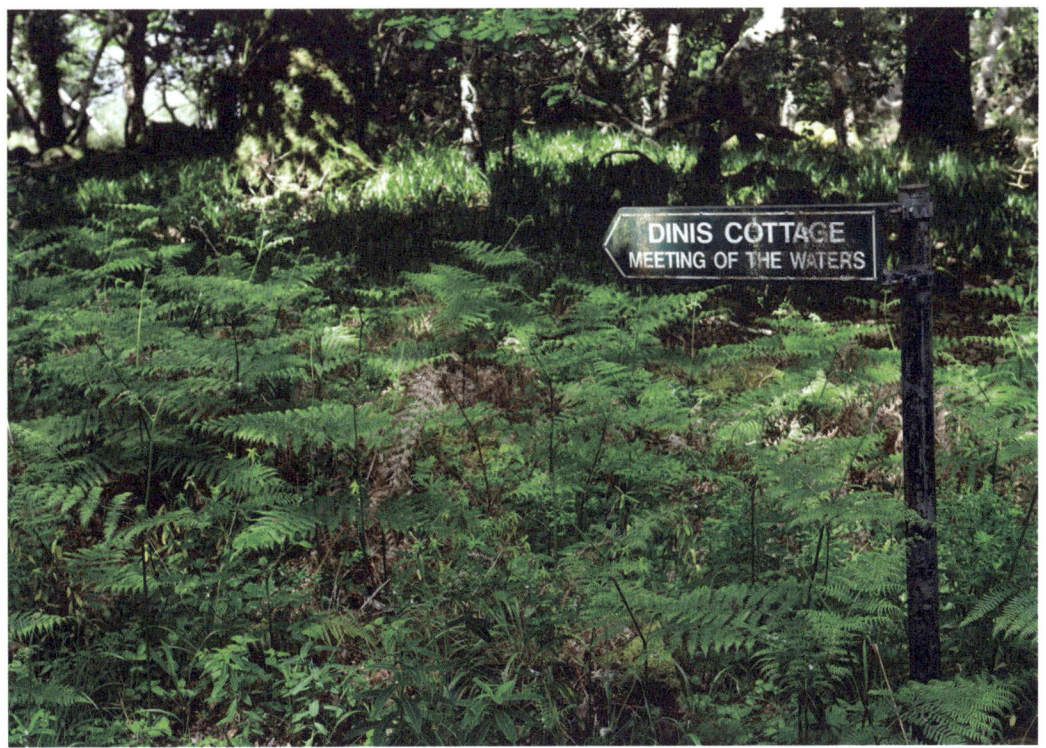

BALLYHOURA NATURE TRAIL, CO. LIMERICK

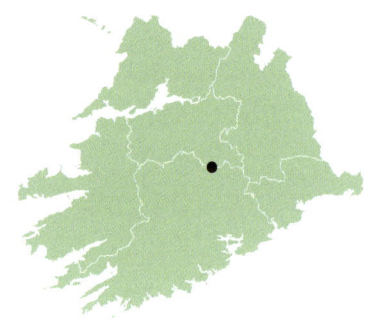

DISTANCE: 2KM

DIFFICULTY: EASY

TIME: 1 HOUR

I am always amazed that more people haven't been to Ballyhoura. It is an incredible facility for runners, hikers and mountain bikers. I spent a lot of time here in my thirties when I was mountain biking and adventure racing. The car park has showers, a coffee shop and bike rental, the walks are mapped and trail marked and the car park is monitored too, so it's really safe.

There are so many walks to choose from, but this one will suit everyone – it's a lovely nature walk for families and a great introduction to the area. Starting at the Ballyhoura Mountain Bike Centre, the Ballyhoura Nature Trail is a family-friendly woodland walk. There is a kids' challenge to spot over twenty creatures that are hidden in the woods – keep your eyes peeled along the 2km trail! Red markers will keep you on the right path.

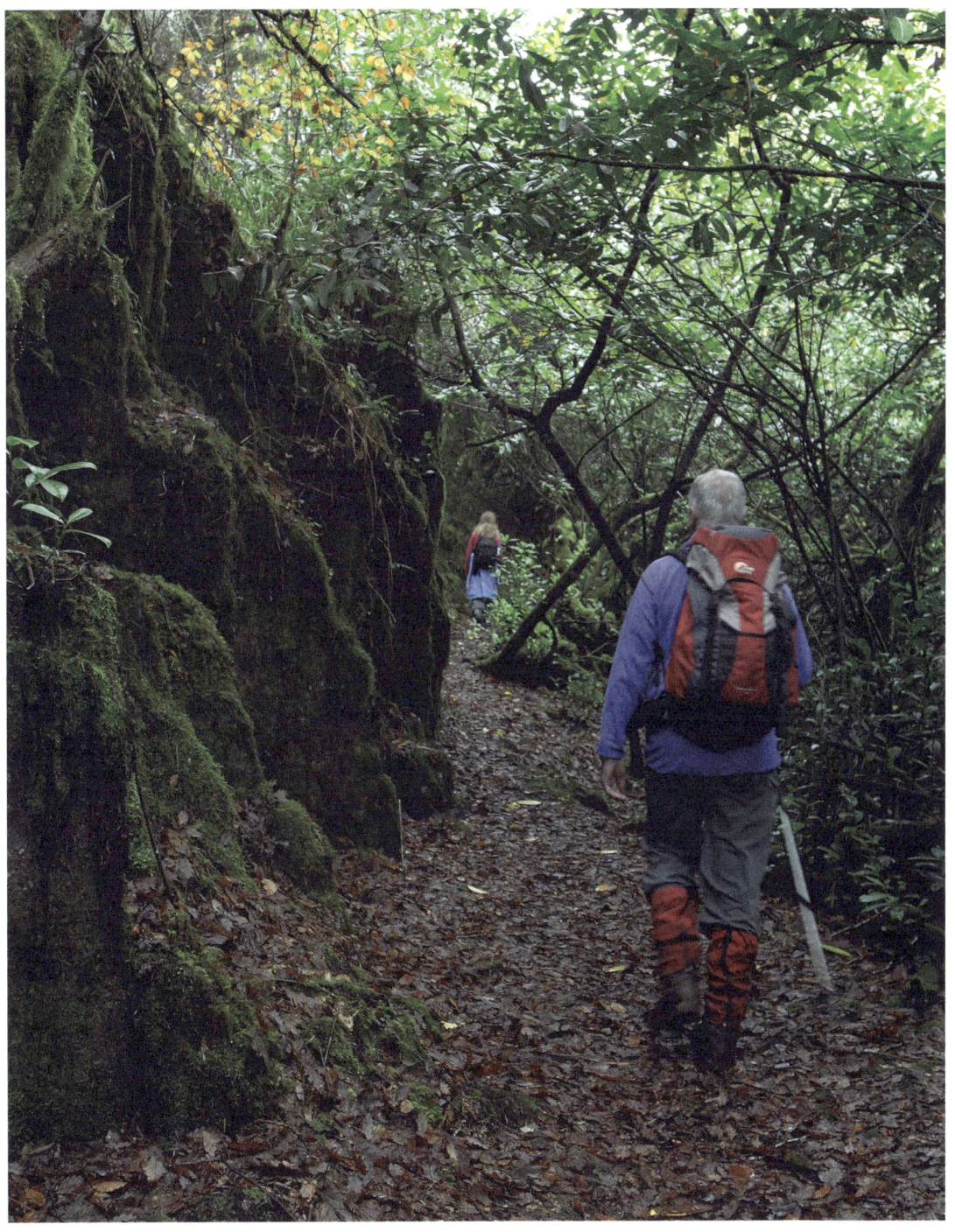

CLIFFS OF MOHER COASTAL WALK, CO. CLARE

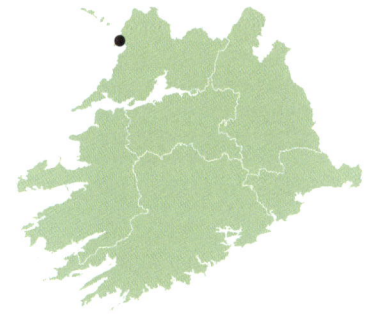

DISTANCE: 8–14KM

DIFFICULTY: MODERATE

TIME: 3–4 HOURS

On a sunny day, this has to be one of the most scenic areas in Ireland. On a wild, windy day, you can barely open the car door! From the Cliffs of Moher, on a clear day, you can see the Aran Islands and Galway Bay, as well as the Twelve Pins and the Maumturk mountains in Connemara, Loop Head to the south and the Dingle Peninsula and Blasket Islands in Kerry. You can make this walk as long or as short as you want, but do give it a go.

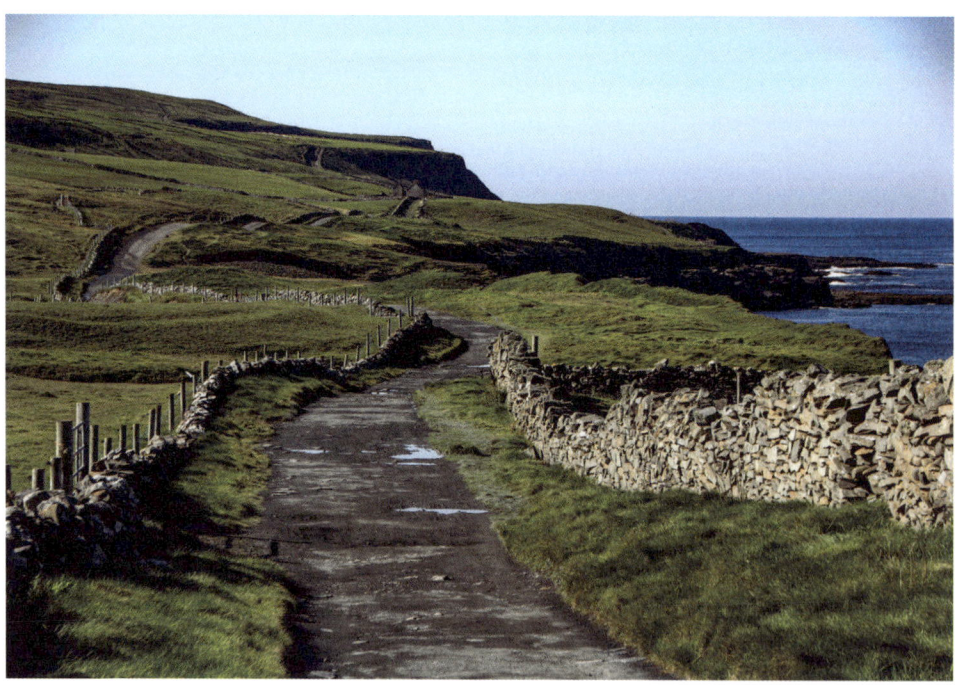

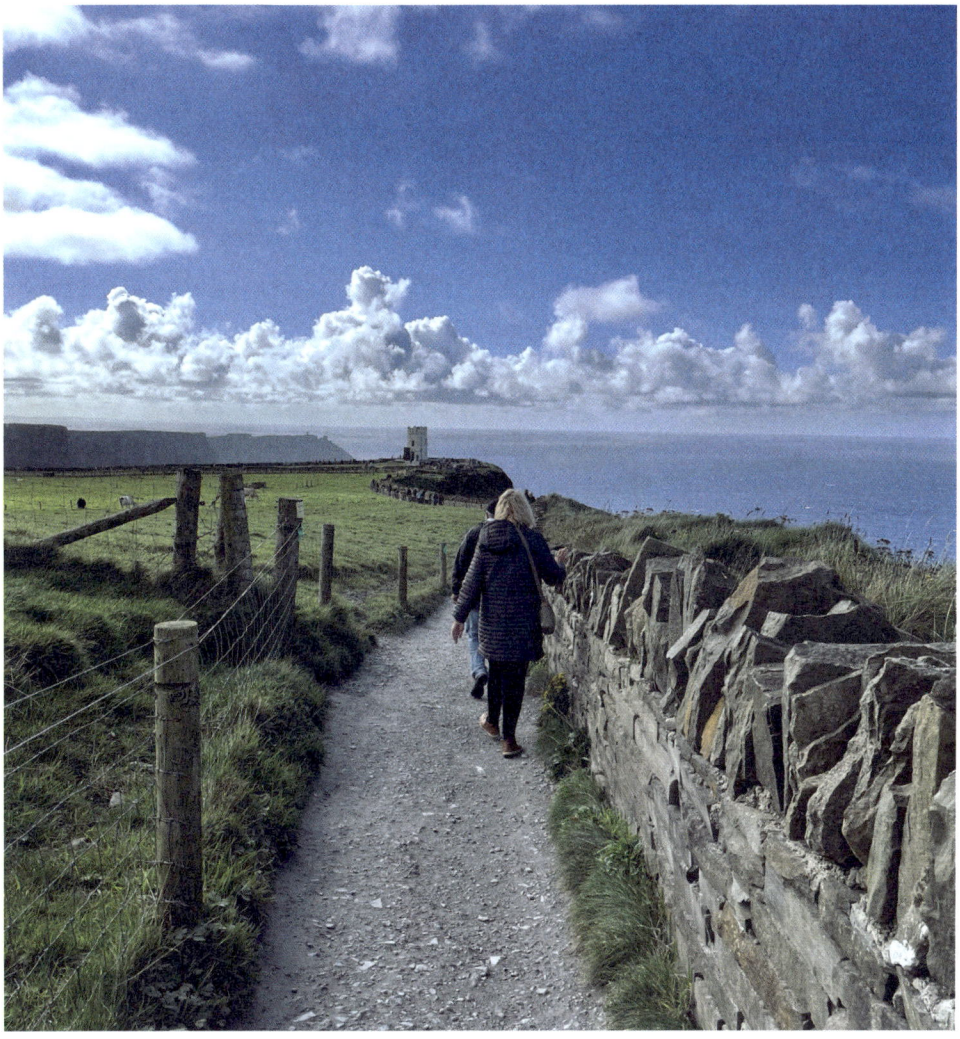

The Cliffs of Moher Coastal Walk is a trail between the villages of Doolin and Liscannor. The walk takes around four hours along a gravel path and you can start in either Liscannor or Doolin. At Liscannor you can park in the town or at the trailhead; the walk finishes at the Cliffs of Moher Visitor Centre, where public transport is available, or you can walk back after fuelling up. Another option is to start in Doolin, from Fisher Street, walk the 8km to the Visitor Centre, and then take the shuttle bus back to Doolin. Or you could walk the entire 14 km along the cliffs all the way to Liscannor. It is a challenging walk, with plenty of steep inclines and declines, so make sure you are prepared, especially if you are going to attempt the longer trail.

DERRYNANE LOOP, CO. KERRY

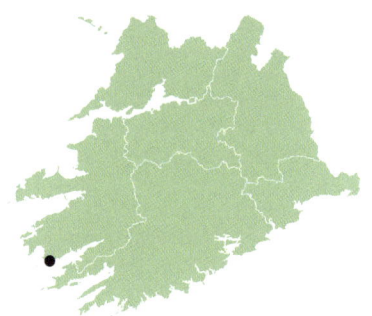

DISTANCE: 8KM

DIFFICULTY: EASY

TIME: 2.5 HOURS

This is a really nice walk on mixed terrain, and it's one for the family too. Bring some snacks with you and take in the countryside views.

The start and end point of the trail is the car park at Derrynane House. From there, walk east and then turn off to the right for the Seashore Nature Trail. Your other option is to go through the metal gate in the south-west corner of the car park, head towards the dunes and then head along the mown grass path. From here you should follow waymarkers showing a yellow arrow and a walker. These markers will guide you all the way back to Derrynane House. As this walk passes through sections of farmland with livestock, dogs are not allowed. It can also get a bit mucky, so it's advisable to wear trail shoes or boots.

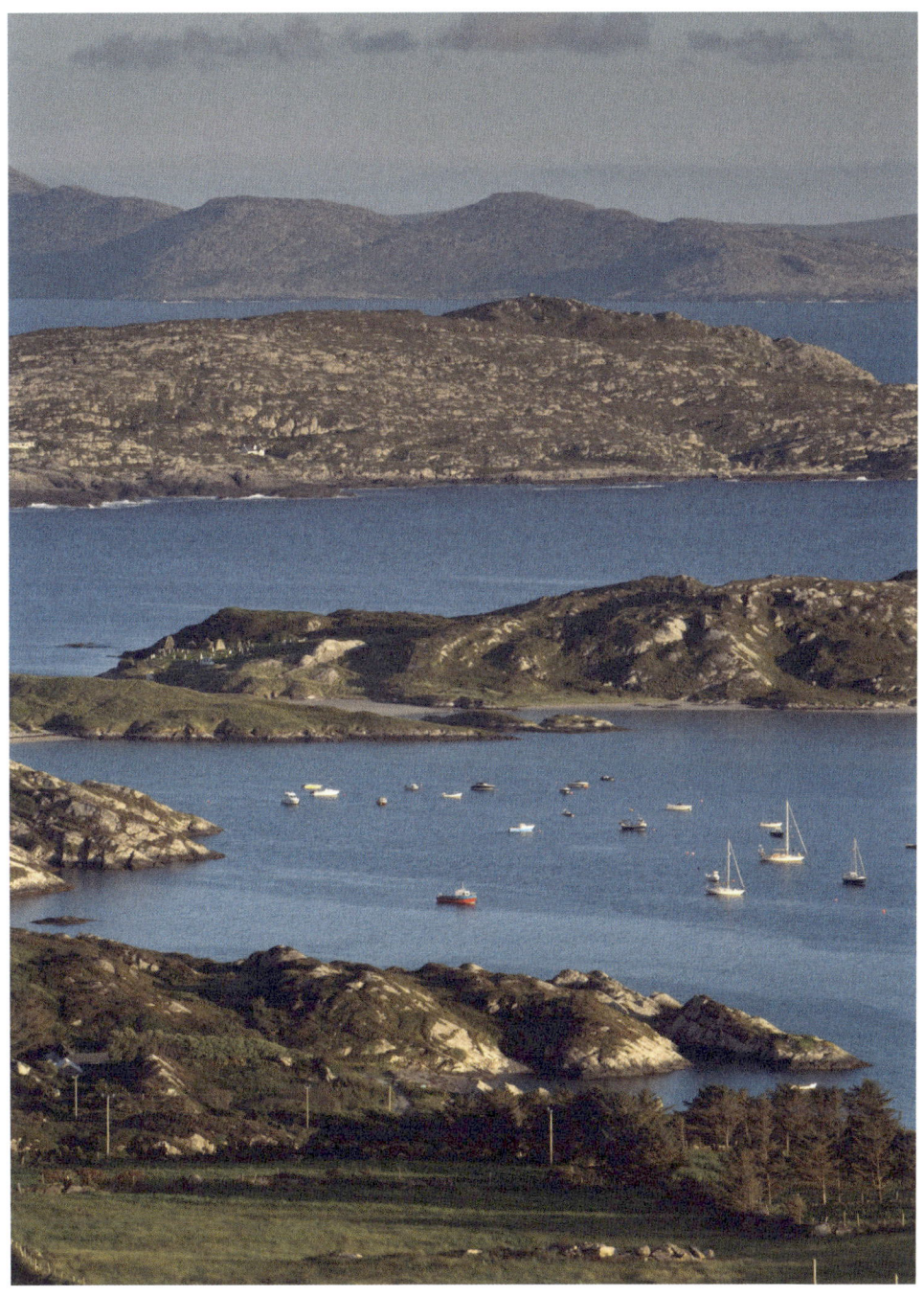

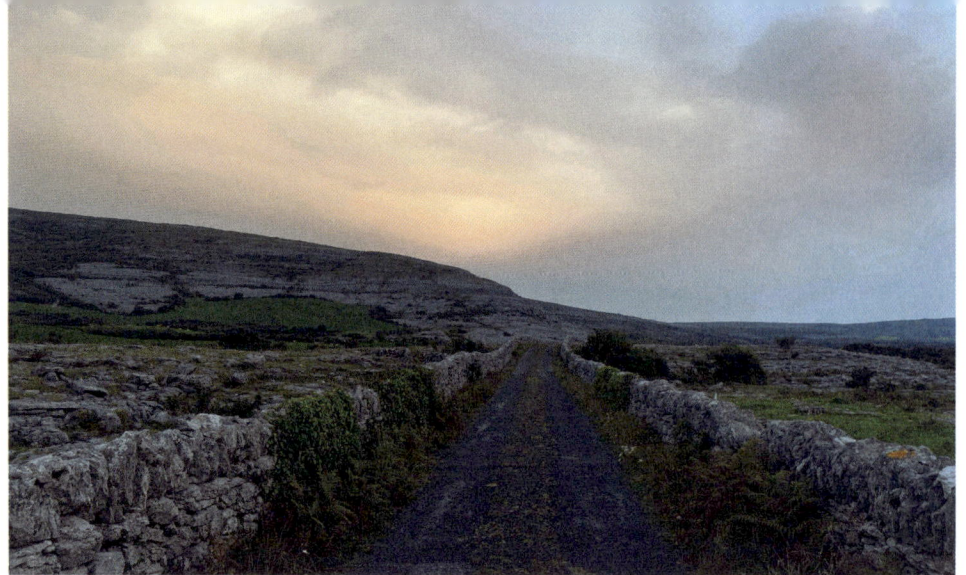

BALLYVAUGHAN WOOD LOOP, CO. CLARE

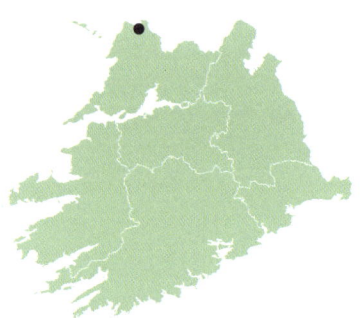

DISTANCE: 8KM

DIFFICULTY: EASY

TIME: 2 HOURS

The walk at Ballyvaughan Wood takes in minor roads, surfaced and sandy roads, green lanes, lush woodland and cross-country terrain. Generally, you'll be able to walk it in runners or trail shoes, but on a very rainy day, or if the ground is wet, you should put on your boots.

Starting at Ballyvaughan's seafront, the walk will take you past thatched cottages, over bridges and stiles, through open fields and farmland, and – at the midpoint – leads you by Aillwee Caves.

These are the Burren's most well known ancient marvel. They boast more than 1km of passages leading into the heart of the mountain, as well as enormous stalagmites and stalactites. You can go for a guided tour if you'd like a break during your walk.

Then back on the road and follow the trails back to Ballyvaughan village where you can enjoy some well-deserved refreshments.

ALLIHIES, CO. CORK

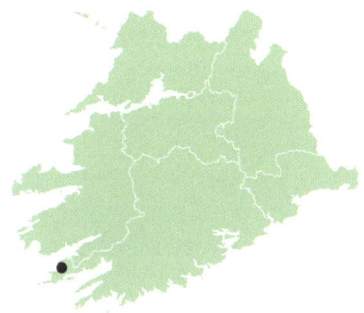

DISTANCE: 7KM

DIFFICULTY: MODERATE

DURATION: 2–3 HOURS

The colourful village of Allihies is the perfect base for exploring some of west Cork's best walking routes, and this one, which sweeps in a loop around the coast, doesn't disappoint. Bird-flecked cliffs, rocky fields, crashing waves and vast sea views mark the coastal part of the walk, which then detours inland. Passing farm buildings, the route climbs up into the disused Mountain Mine area, which reveals Allihies' past as a copper-mining hub in the nineteenth century. Keep going and you'll eventually loop back to the village, where music, food and pints await inside the bright red O'Neill's Bar & Restaurant.

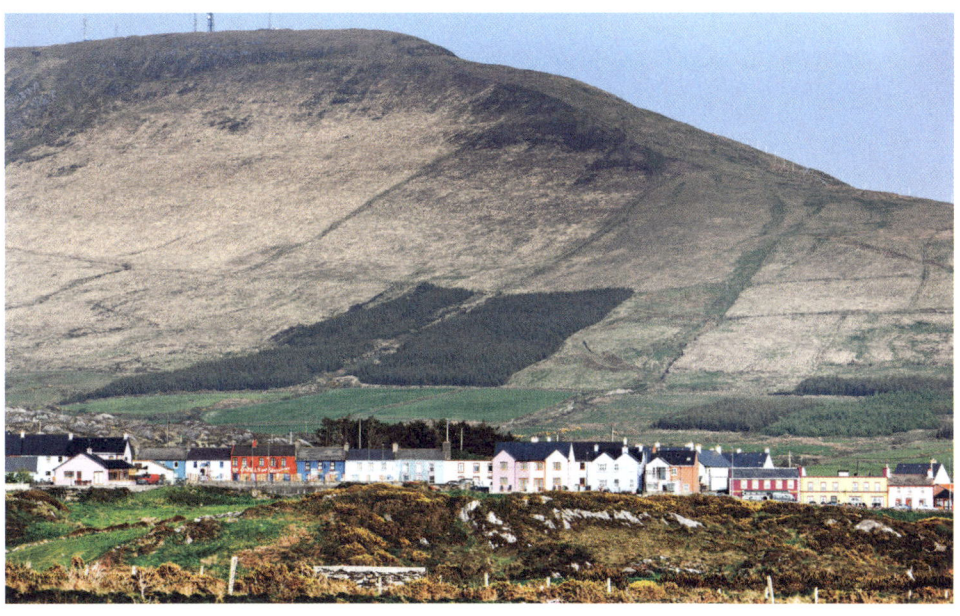

CONNACHT

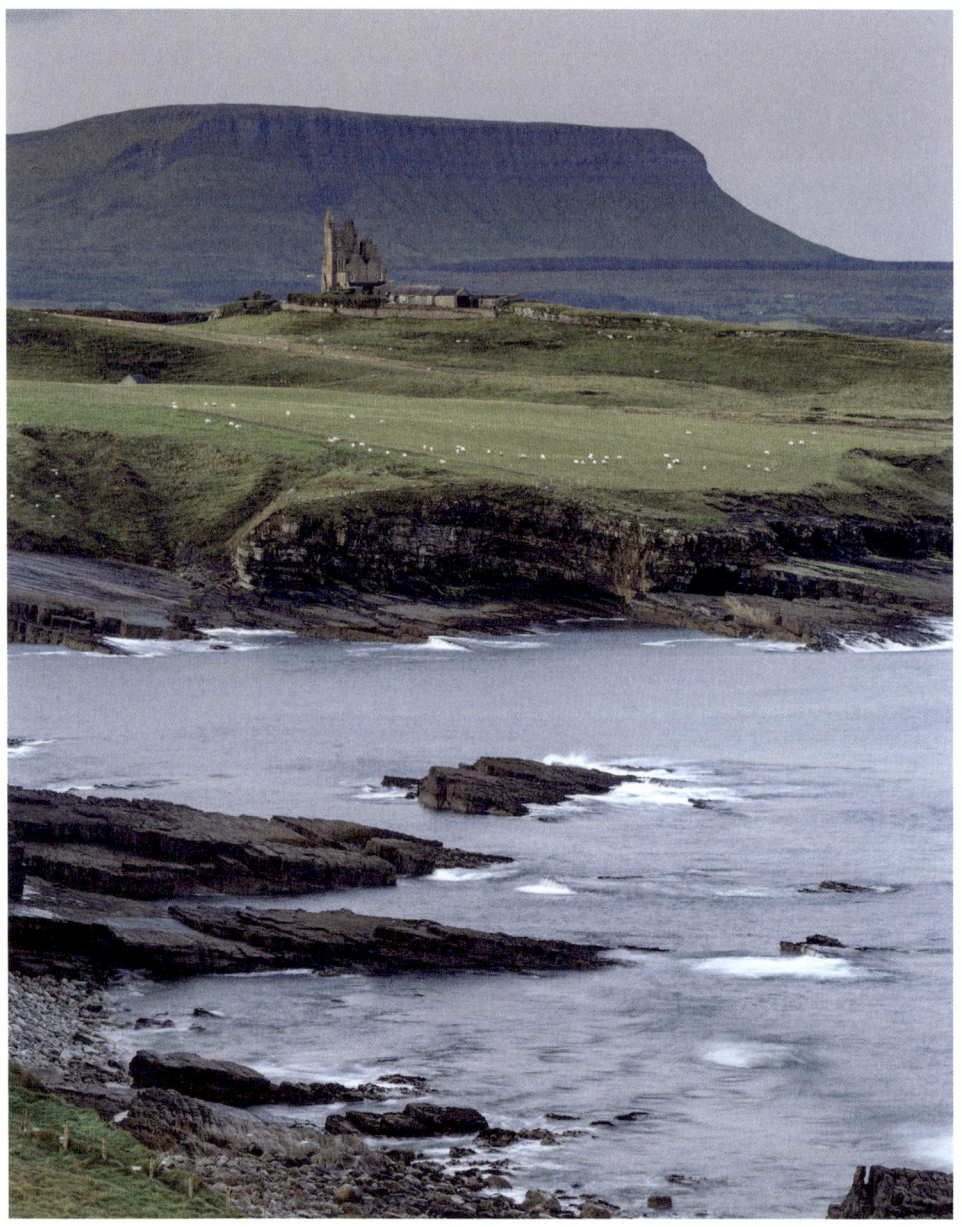

MULLAGHMORE HEAD, CO. SLIGO

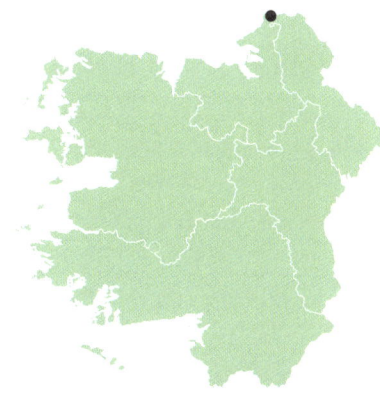

DISTANCE: 6KM

DIFFICULTY: EASY

TIME: 1.5 HOURS

Sligo has so many walking and hiking routes, catering for all fitness levels. This lovely scenic walk will suit all fitness types, and families too. It consists of a mixture of footpaths, off-road walking trails and public roads, and provides incredible panoramic views of Donegal Bay and Slieve League beyond, as well as Benbulben and the Dartry Mountains, so there is lots to see, and lots to keep the family entertained. Please remember to follow the rules of walking on the road, and walk against the traffic whenever you can.

The best place to park is in Mullaghmore village, at the seafront. Starting your walk, keep the harbour on your right and take the road out of the village that passes the Pier Head Hotel. There are a couple of steep sections, and do take care when walking past unguarded parts of the road where the cliff falls away. This walk is a loop, so you'll end up coming back into the village from the opposite side.

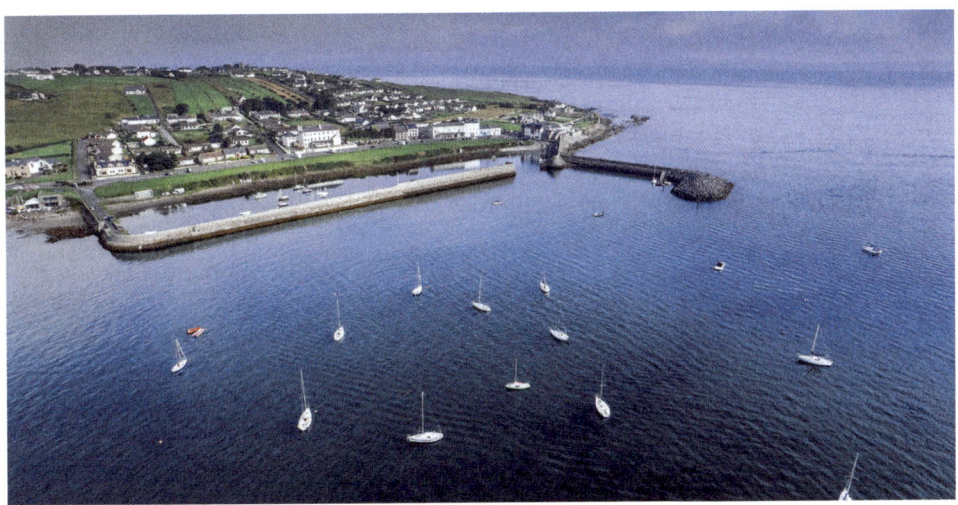

DIAMOND HILL FROM LETTERFRACK, CO. GALWAY

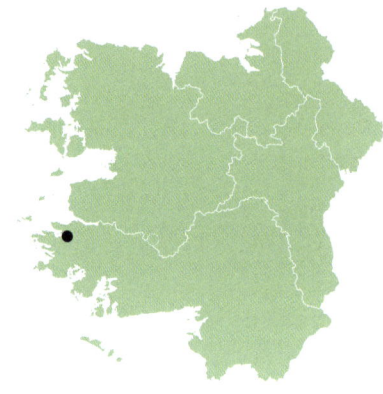

DISTANCE: 3KM–3.7KM

DIFFICULTY: EASY TO MODERATE

TIME: 45 MINUTES–2 HOURS

I love Connemara and I have spent so much time there racing and hill-walking over the years. This walk is in the Connemara National Park, beside the village of Letterfrack. Diamond Hill stands at 442 metres high – whether the walk is easy or moderate depends on the option you choose. Both walks start at the visitors' centre, where you can also park.

There are two walks here to choose from: the 3km Lower Diamond Walk, and the 3.7km Upper Diamond Walk. Both walks are suitable for all levels and no special equipment is required, but in autumn or winter I would recommend proper footwear and a good rain jacket as it can get really cold and windy towards the top. Both routes are very well signposted, and gravel footpaths and wooden boardwalks guide you over the bog as you approach the mountain. Near the foot of the mountain, you can continue walking the Lower Diamond Walk or turn to tackle the Upper Diamond Walk. There is a steady climb to the summit but the magnificent view is worth it. In fact, the views on both these walks are second to none. Diamond Hill looks down on Connemara National Park, Kylemore Abbey, Inishturk and Inishark and the Twelve Pins mountain range. The loop continues down the opposite side of the mountain, where you rejoin the lower walk. If you like, you can also complete that walk, or you can head back to the visitors' centre where you started.

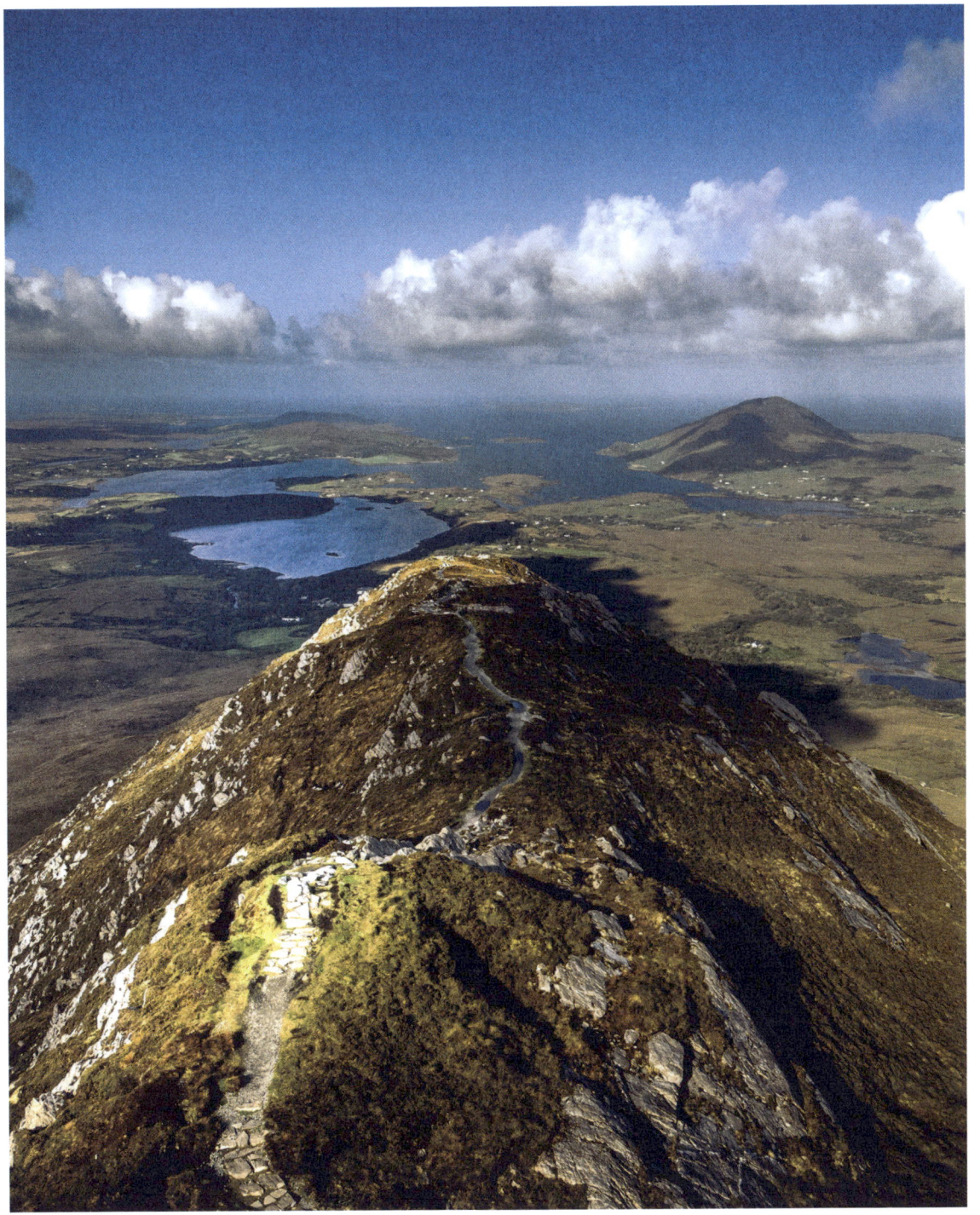

CROAGH PATRICK, CO. MAYO

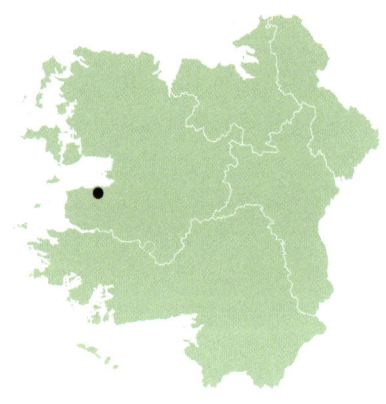

DISTANCE: 8KM

DIFFICULTY: MODERATE

TIME: 4 HOURS

I don't think there is anyone in Ireland who doesn't know Croagh Patrick. The last time I was there was with the epic walk organised by Charlie Bird in 2022, when what seemed like the whole country turned out to support Charlie and his family and take on the climb. It was a very special day with an incredible atmosphere and sense of community, everyone helping each other to the top.

The view from the top is just breathtaking. The walk is challenging in places, but trust me, you will be blown away by the view. Walking up Croagh Patrick is fairly difficult in places as it's steep, there are uneven rocks to get over and the upper slopes have a lot of loose, slippery scree. It has got much better in recent years – a lot of work has been done to improve the path – but I would wear trail runners or boots for this one. I have seen people do it in runners and they aren't ideal.

Starting in the car park at Murrisk, where there is a shop and coffee shop, head to your first landmark after the visitors' centre, which is the statue of St Patrick that was erected in 1928. You'll walk through a small gate and then the upward climb begins fairly quickly.

The easiest way to approach the walk is to split it into three sections. The first section takes you from the car park to the shelf of the mountain. The initial slope is fairly reasonable but gets steep in places and the surface is grassy and rocky in parts. You'll be rewarded for every step with glorious views out over Clew Bay as you climb.

The second section is not as hard as it takes you along the shoulder of the mountain to the base of the upper slope. It's a gentle recovery after the initial hard work and then it preps you for the final section.

The final section is the start of a huge pyramid-shaped mountain top covered in loose scree, which makes for tough climbing and slippery conditions. You'll need to be careful along this steep section, and sometimes walking in a side-to-side or zig-zag motion can make it a little easier on the legs and the lungs. But remember, walking isn't a race. Take your time, take a break if you need to and take in the views. As you approach the summit you will see the small church and on your right you will see the incredible panoramic views around south Mayo and the islands of Clew Bay that make this hike so worthwhile. The top of the mountain is big enough to walk around and to sit and enjoy a sandwich or a cup of tea. It can get cold up there, so don't hang around too long, and make sure you have plenty of layers on to prevent you getting too cold.

On the way back down, take it easy and again split it into three sections, taking your time and not rushing it.

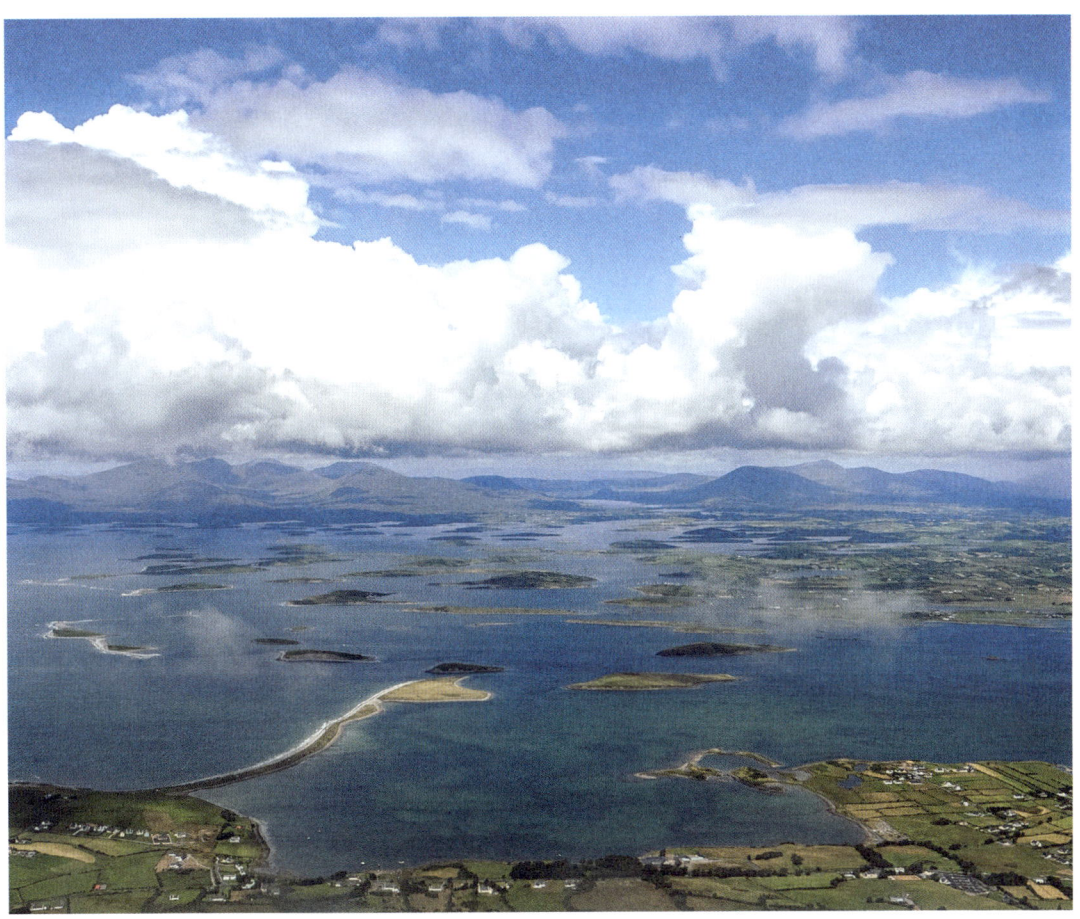

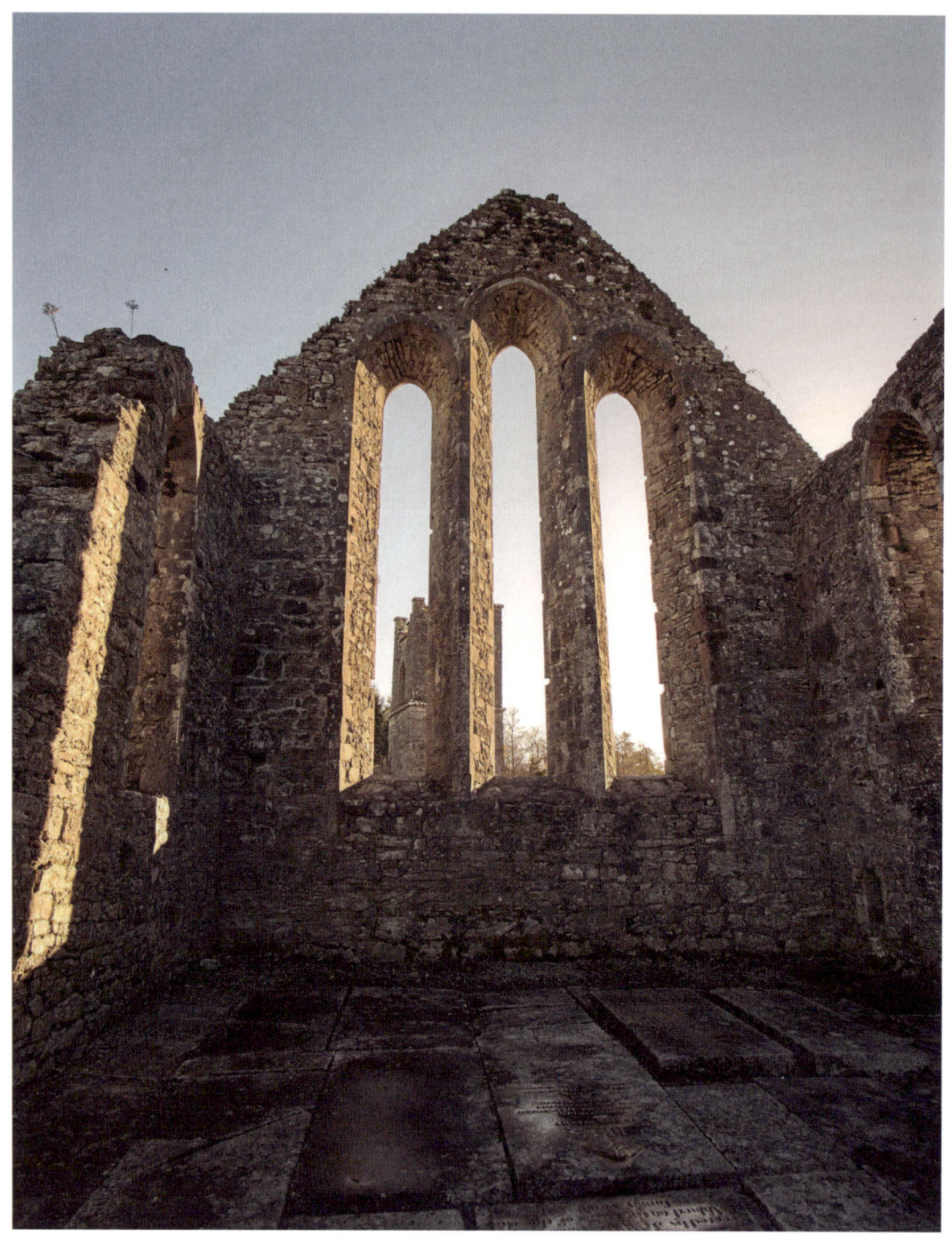

CONG WOODS, CO. MAYO

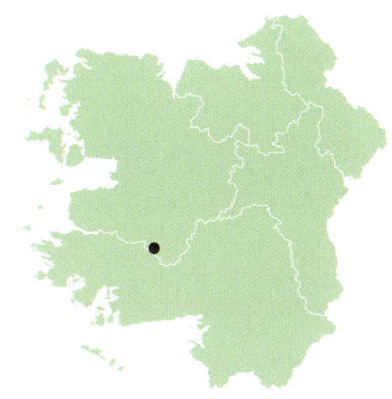

DISTANCE: 6KM

DIFFICULTY: EASY

TIME: 1.5 HOURS

This is a really lovely, easy walk suitable for all the family. Starting at the church car park, enter the Cong Abbey grounds across the road and walk through the yew grove on the grounds. Cross the Cong River on the small stone bridge, the Abbey Bridge. At the far side of the bridge, go into the forest through a stone gateway. Turn left along the path for about 200 metres. Then turn right and follow the nature trail markers.

At the finger sign for Teach Aille (Cliff House in English), turn right and go down into the cave site. Steps beside the cave lead to higher ground above the cave. Follow the marked trail to a junction. Here, turn left under a viaduct, which is on the Cong/Cornamona road. Proceed along the trail to an old disused house on your left. Turn right here and walk towards Pigeon Hole Cave. There are steps down into the cave, where you can see a stream that flows underground from Lough Mask into Lough Corrib. From here, head along the track leading back to Cong. You will pass under a small viaduct and along the banks of the Cong River and back to Abbey Bridge, then cross back into the Cong Abbey grounds, where you began.

PORTUMNA FOREST PARK, CO. GALWAY

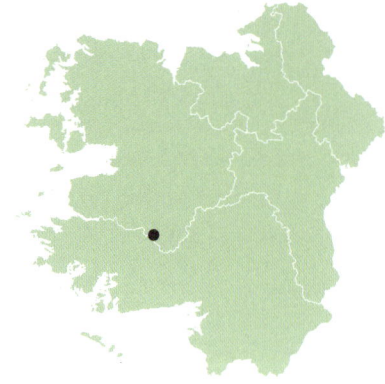

DISTANCE: 4–10 KM

DIFFICULTY: EASY

TIME: UP TO 3 HOURS

There are lots and lots of trails in Portumna Forest Park. Many are family-friendly and many have gravelled or tarred forest road surfaces, along with some wide timber boardwalks. One of the best things about the trails here is that they are generally on the flat with very little gradient, making them accessible for buggies and kids' bikes.

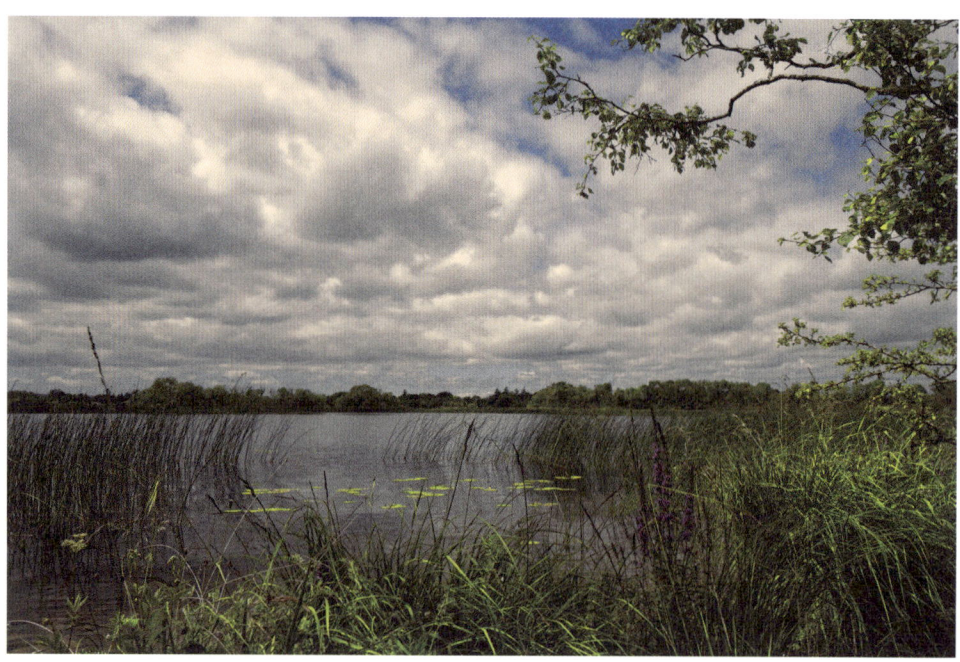

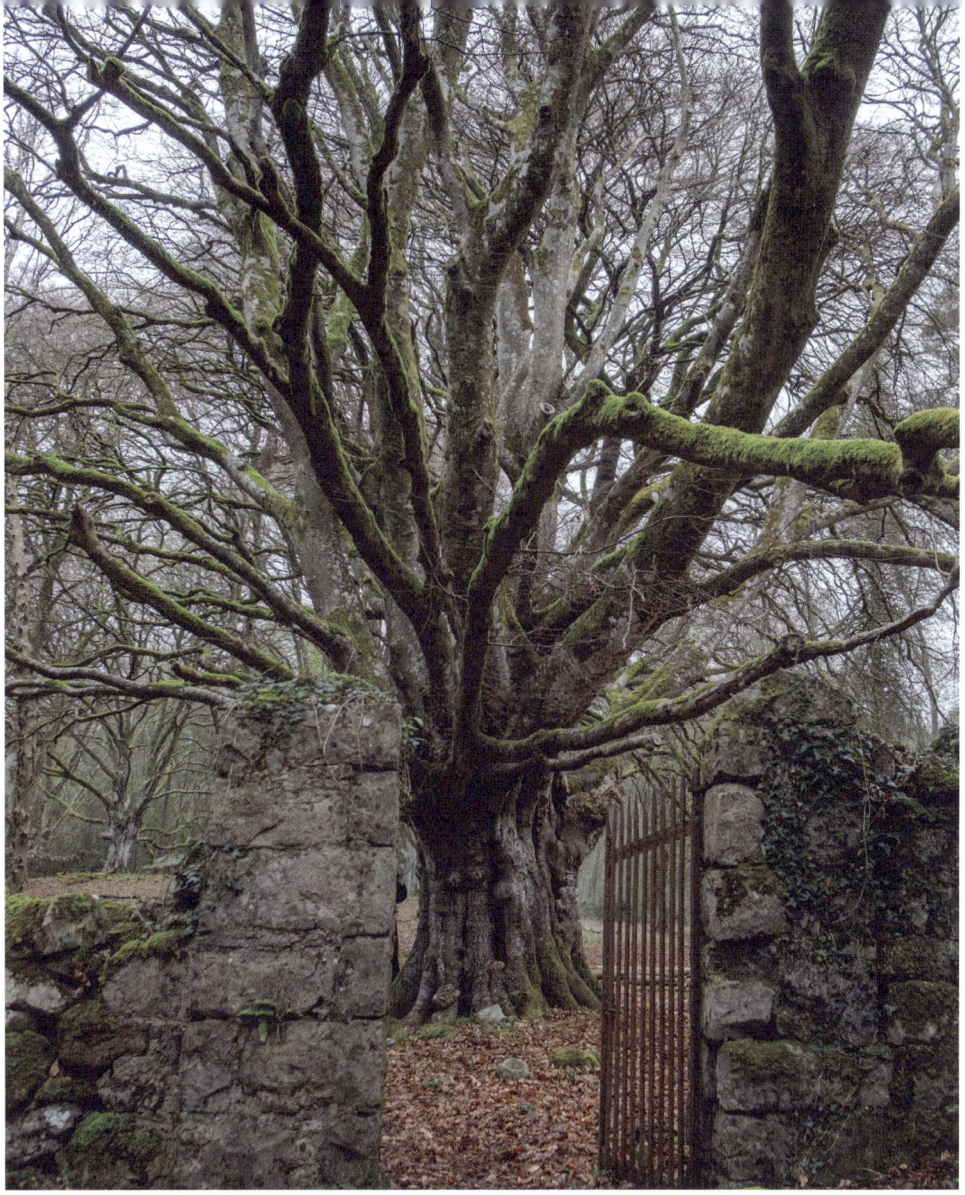

When you park up, you can choose between walks from 30 minutes to three hours, and all are doable for all fitness levels. The trails are all marked and signposted and there are some great family nature trail options too. Another bonus is that there is plenty of car parking, plus toilet facilities are available on site and it is a really safe place to walk.

INISHBOFIN WESTQUARTER LOOP, CO. GALWAY

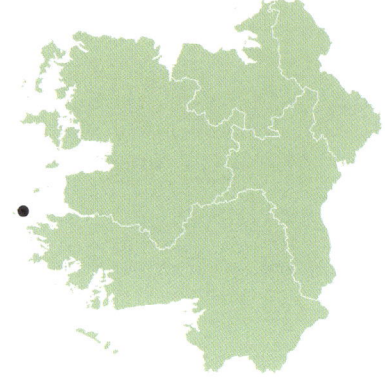

DISTANCE: 5KM

DIFFICULTY: EASY

DURATION: 2 HOURS

Catch the ferry from Cleggan pier in Connemara and travel over to the small island of Inishbofin, which sits 8km out in the Atlantic. Much of the island is an Area of Special Conservation, which makes walking here extra special. Starting at the pier, the Westquarter Loop leads around the western part of the island, past blowholes and sea arches, cliffs, a beach and the remains of an Iron Age promontory fort. It's an invigorating walk with great Atlantic views and gives a real sense of escape. Heading back to Bofin Harbour, drop into the Inishbofin House Hotel for a late lunch in the bar before catching the ferry back to Cleggan.

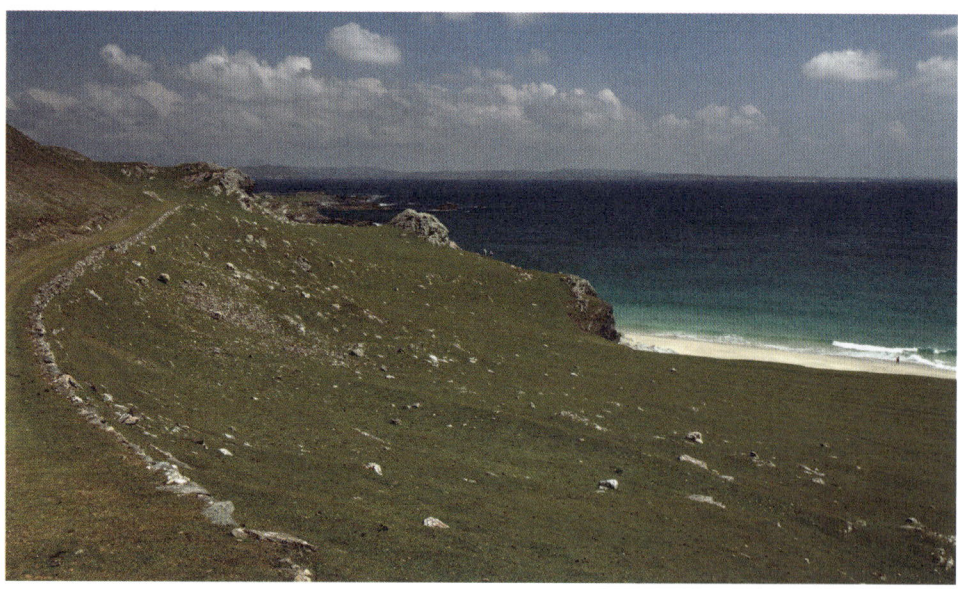

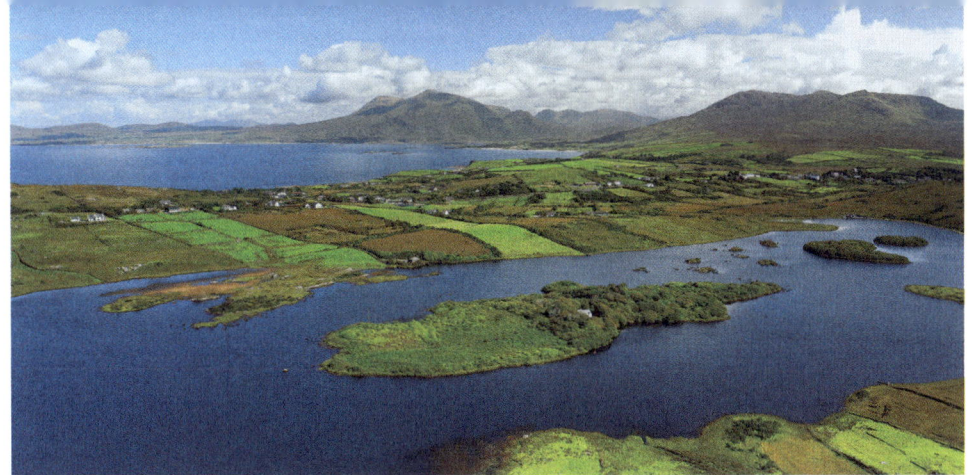

MWEELREA, CO. MAYO

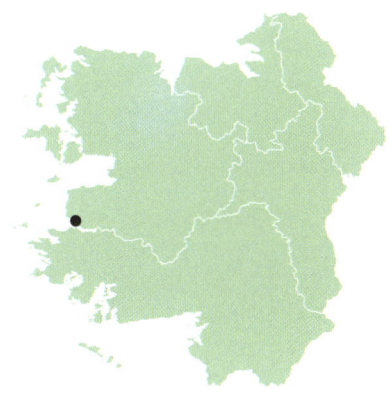

DISTANCE: 11KM

DIFFICULTY: HARD

TIME: 5 HOURS

Now this is a tough one. Of the four tallest peaks, I find Mweelrea the most challenging. The ground is boggy and tiring and the weather can change here really quickly, so it is a walk I would only do with a guide. There are several routes to the summit, but none of the options is marked with signage. The directions below will take you to the summit via the Silver Strand route, the only route I have walked.

You have two options for parking if you're hiking this route. You can either park at the Silver Strand beach car park and walk 1km to the start of the trail. Or, if parking is available, you can park at the bottom of the lane beside the gate just off the road. It is fairly remote, so don't leave any valuables in your car. The trail starts when you enter the gate. You'll need to cross the stream and make your way straight up towards the gully. When you reach the shoulder, you will see a trail to take you to the summit, and you come back down via the same route. Twice when I have been up here with a guide a thick blanket of cloud has come in and I was very glad to have the guide with me! This route is roughly an 11km round trip, with some beautiful views to reward your hard work.

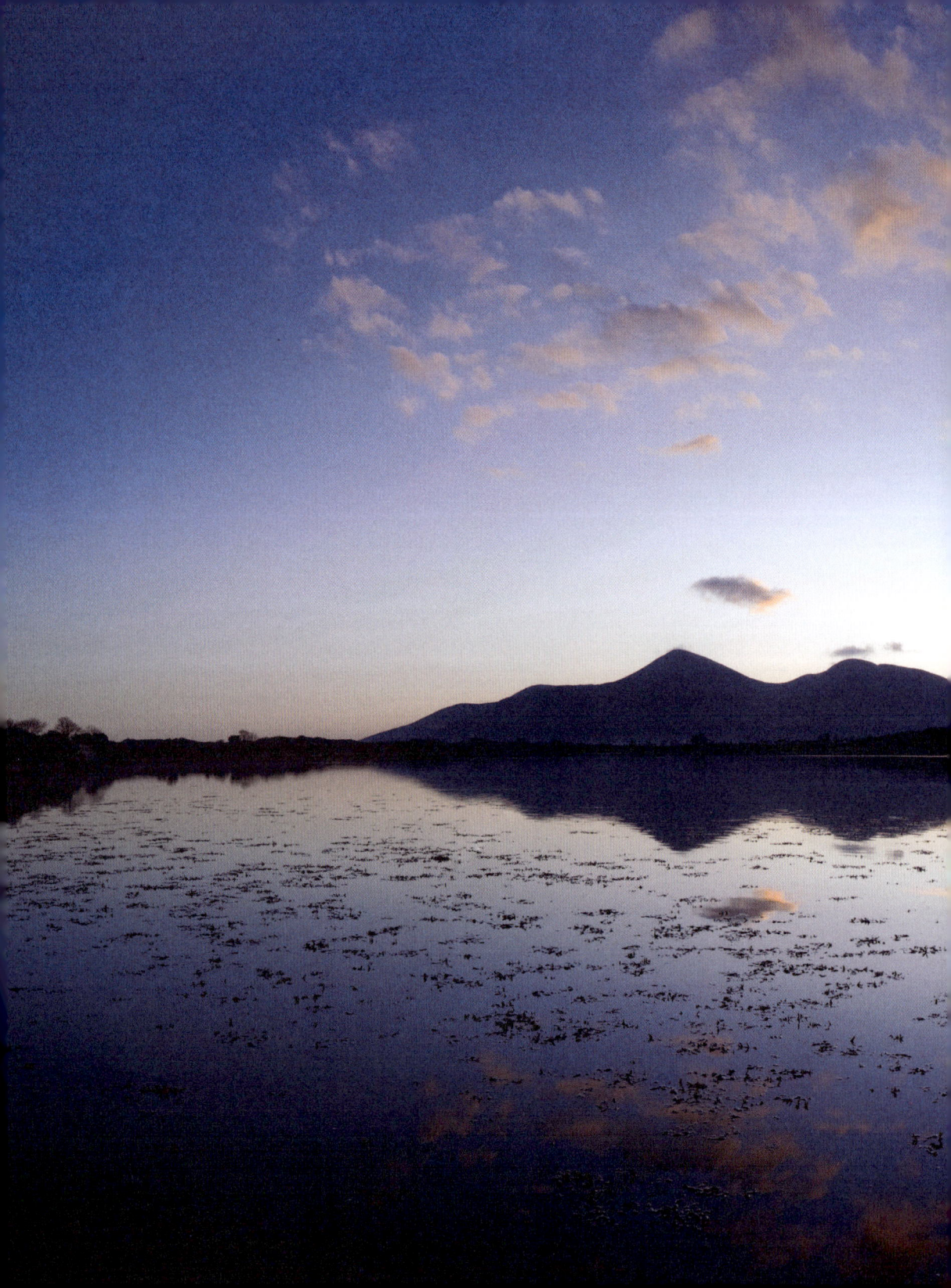

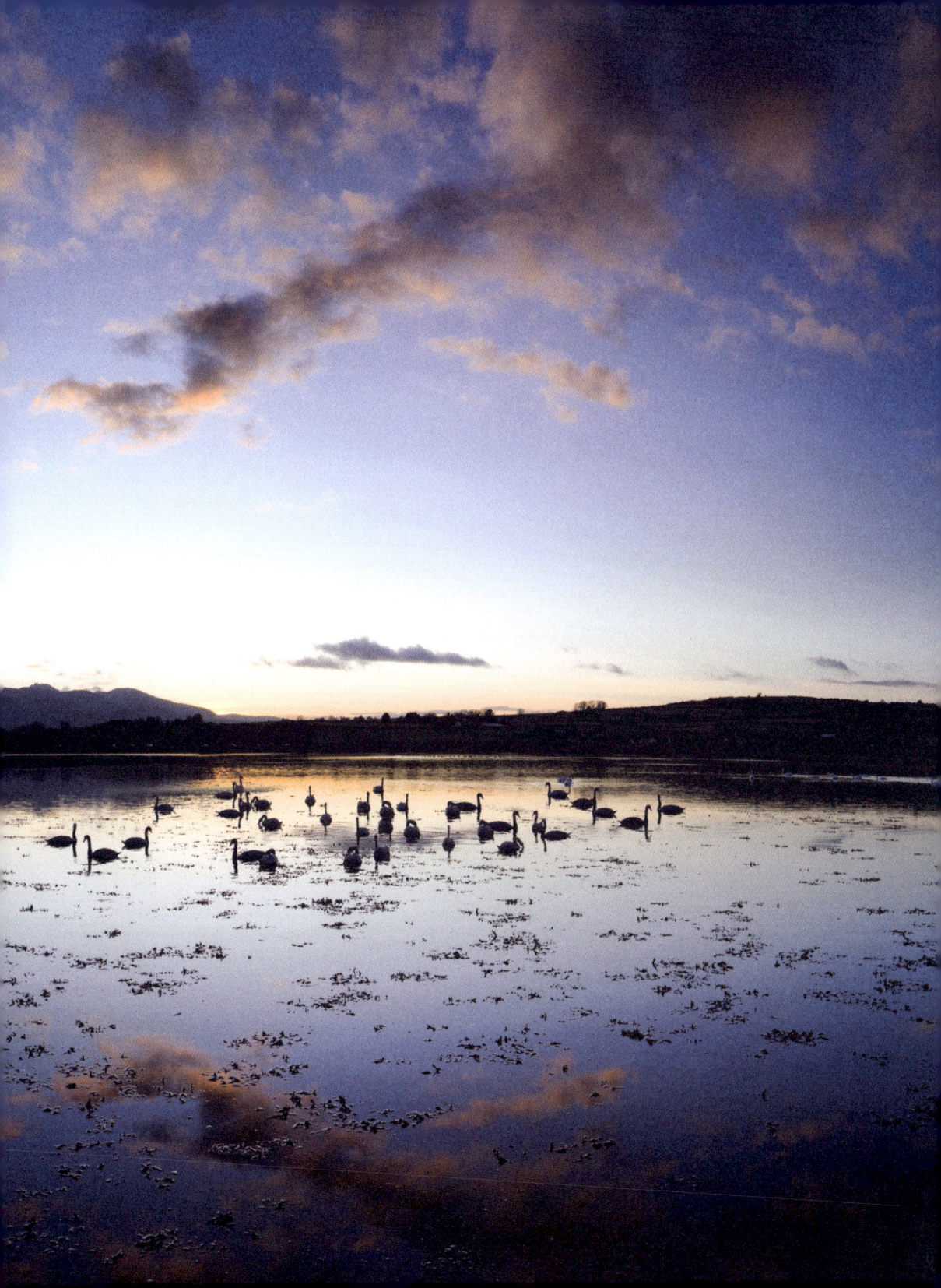

ULSTER

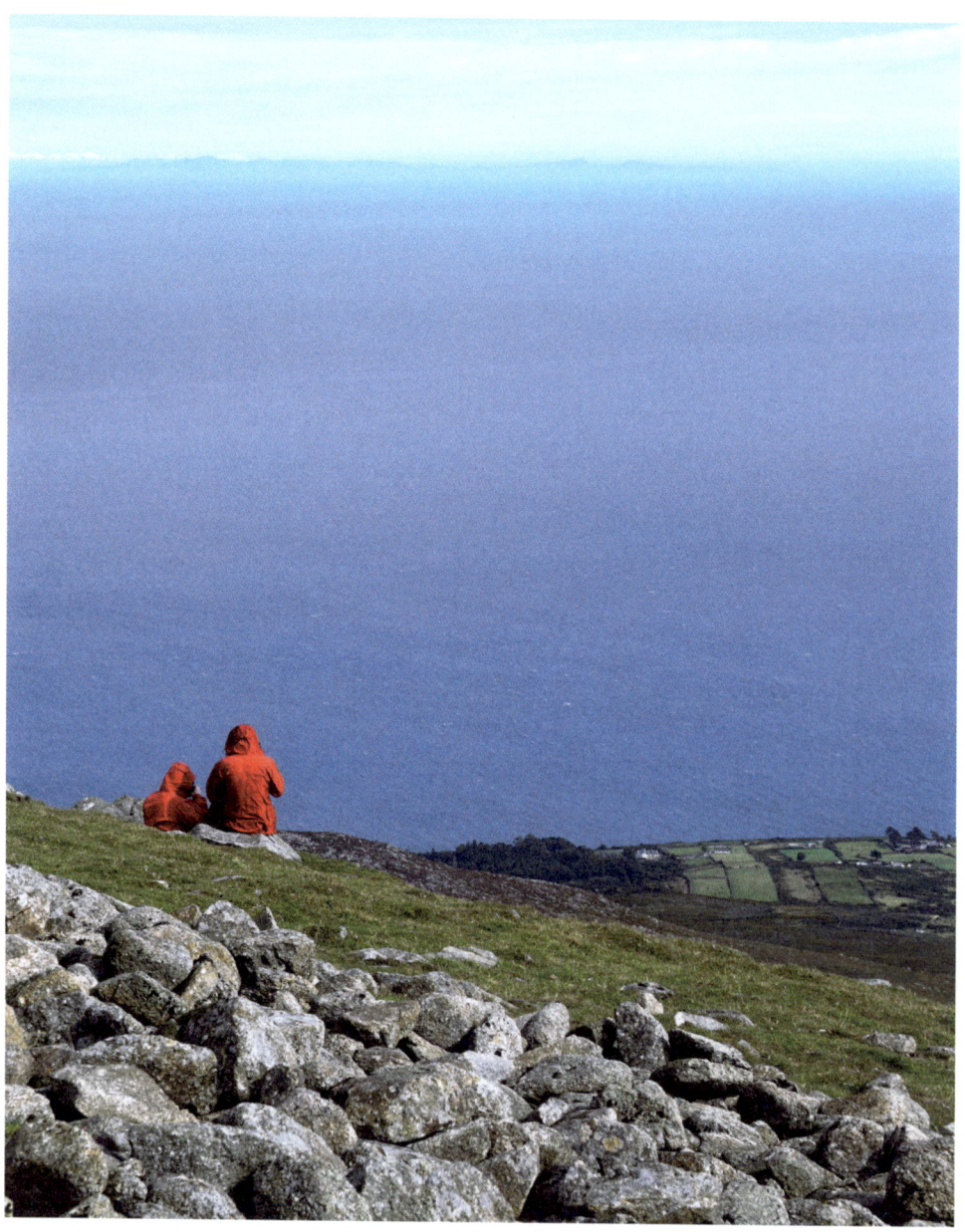

SLIEVE DONARD, CO. DOWN

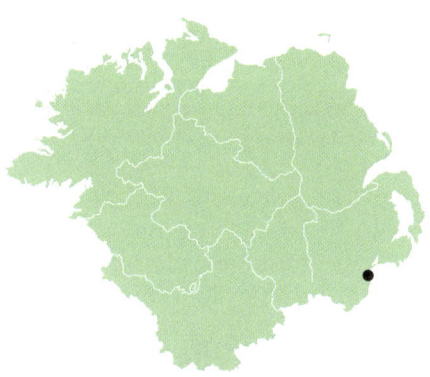

DISTANCE: 9–9.5KM

DIFFICULTY: HARD

TIME: 5–6 HOURS

Slieve Donard is the highest peak in the Mournes, and the walk up it is another of my favourites. Historic, scenic, challenging but doable, it isn't as far from Dublin as you might think – around a two-hour drive; and the second hour has some beautiful scenery as you drive along with the sea on one side and the Mountains of Mourne on the other.

To start with, leave the car park in Donard Park and head towards the mountain. Follow the Glen River uphill through a lovely old woodland of oak, birch and Scots pine. At the bridge – the first of three on this route – cross to the opposite bank.

Continue uphill through the forest, above a river, for about 400m until you reach another bridge. At this point, cross back to the left-hand side of the river and continue uphill through the trees. At the next bridge, continue across the forest road and onto the rough track heading up towards the mountains, with forest on your right, until you reach a gate and stile. Cross the stile and go along the track above the river for about 2km, heading directly up towards the saddle between Donard and Commedagh. From here, the path crosses the river and continues uphill to the saddle, where it meets the Mourne Wall. When you get to the Mourne Wall, turn left and follow the wall towards the summit. It really is steep, so take your time, take your breaks and enjoy the experience along the way.

Descend by the same route, staying close to the wall until you reach the saddle again. Return to Donard Park following the line of the Glen River, the same way you came up. You can then head into Newcastle for some well-deserved food.

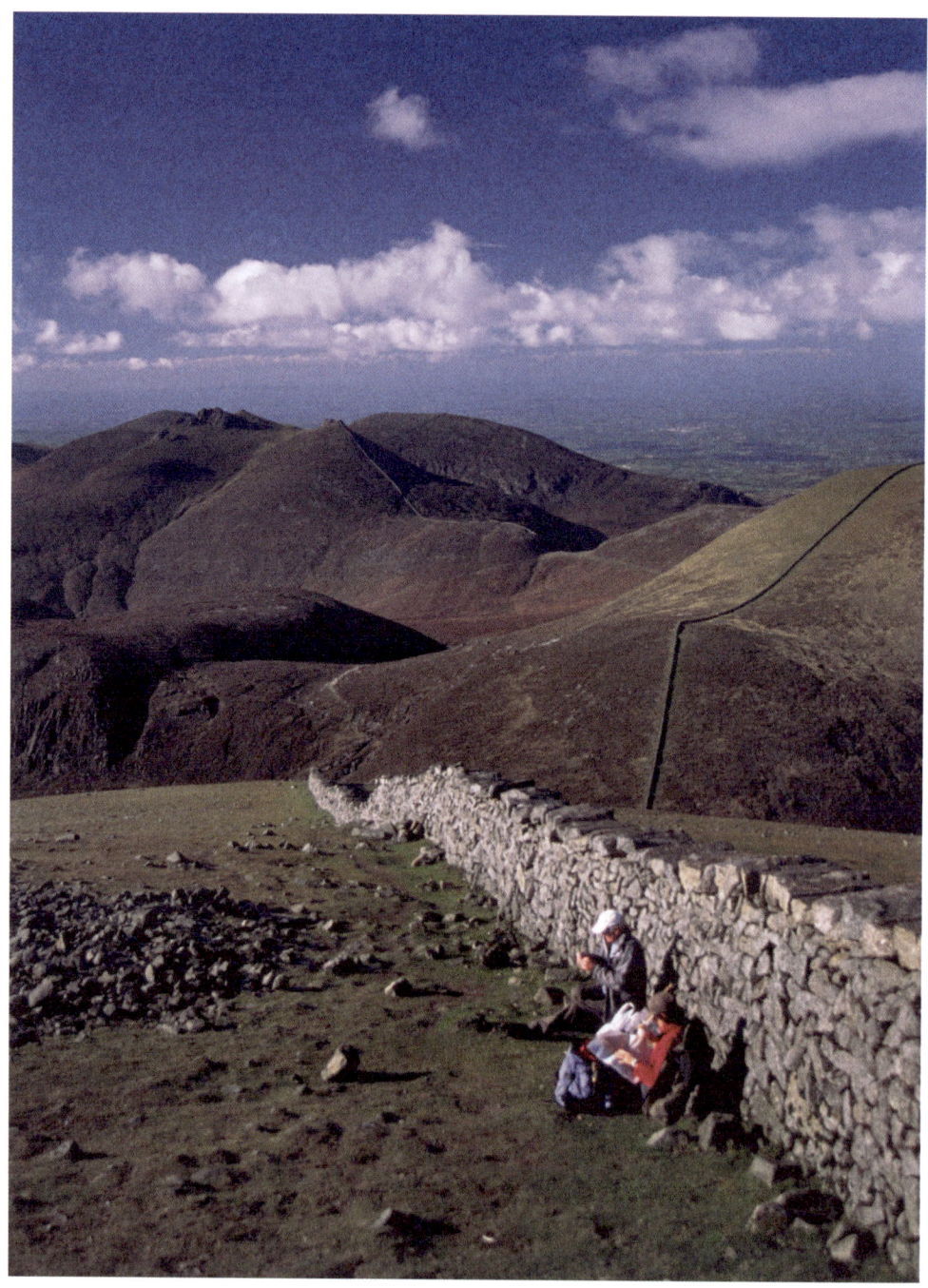

MOURNE MOUNTAINS, CO. DOWN

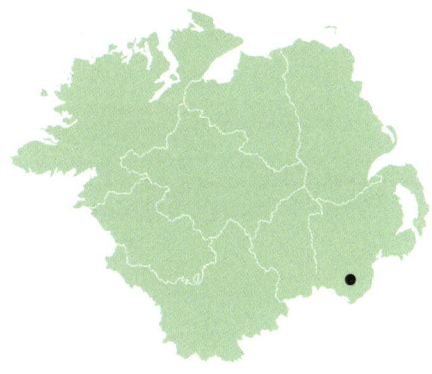

The Mourne Mountains are a walker's paradise and you have so many options to choose from. The website www.walkni.com has great information and maps on all of the walks you can do. I have picked a few out here that you will like.

SLIEVE BINNIAN

DISTANCE: 11KM

DIFFICULTY: EASY

TIME: 2–3 HOURS

This is a fantastic circular walking route that begins at Carrick Little car park near Annalong village and follows the Mourne Wall to the summit of Slieve Binnian. It then traverses between the spectacular South and North Tors before you descend along a track past the Blue Lough and Annalong Forest, before returning to the car park where you started. You'll see some fine panoramas along the way, with the striking Silent Valley and Ben Crom reservoirs below, and towering summits beyond providing dramatic views.

BEARNAGH AND MEELMORE

DISTANCE: 9.5KM

DIFFICULTY: MODERATE

TIME: 4–5 HOURS

This is a more challenging walk. The route takes in the peaks of Slieve Bearnagh and Slieve Meelmore, finishing by leading down Happy Valley and along a section of the Ulster Way. This circuit uses the Mourne Wall as a handrail on the higher parts of the mountain; on a clear day it offers superb views stretching as far as the Sperrins, Lough Neagh and Strangford Lough.

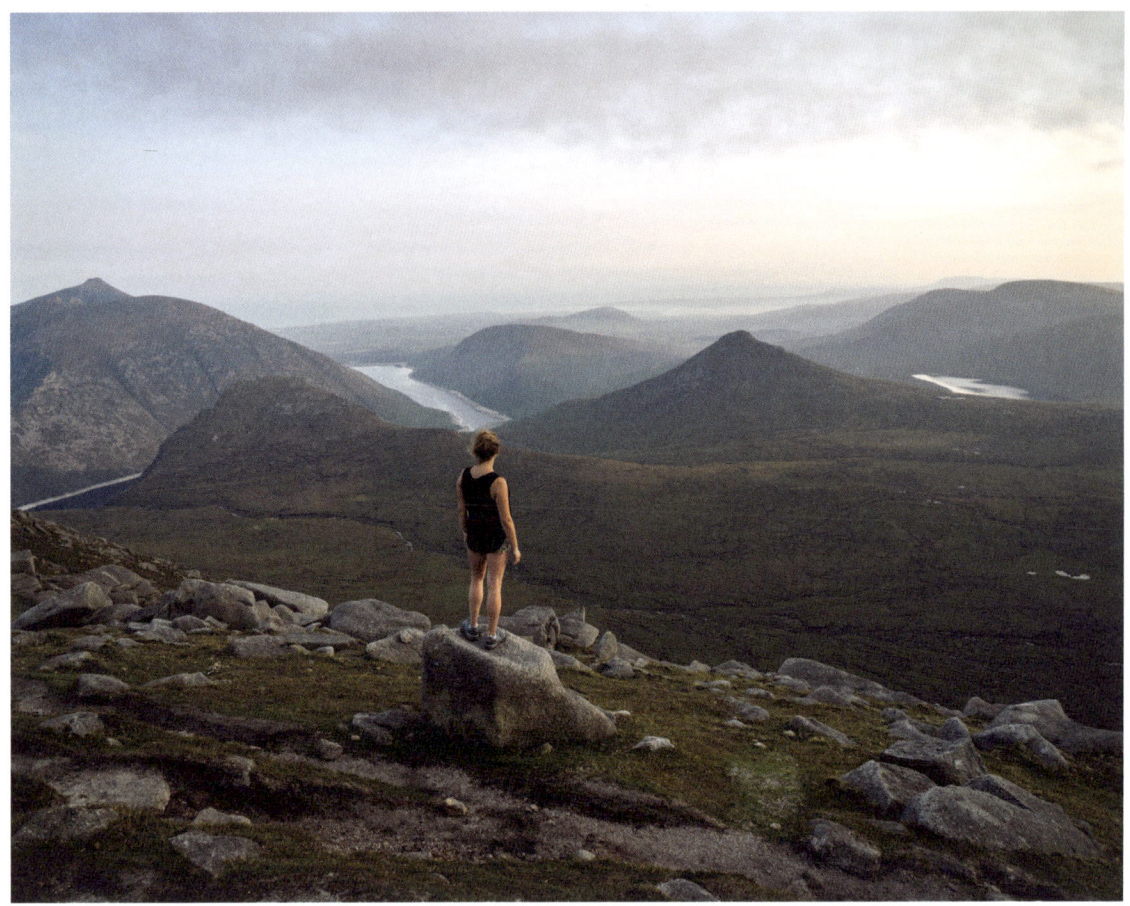

MOURNE WALL CHALLENGE

DISTANCE: 35KM

DIFFICULTY: HARD

TIME: 15 HOURS

This is a very challenging and highly strenuous walk. It follows the 35km (22 miles) of the historic Mourne Wall, and incorporates climbing and descending 15 peaks, including seven of the ten highest mountains in the Mournes and Northern Ireland. Not for the faint-hearted, it is sure to reward you with a truly unique experience.

HEN, COCK AND PIGEON ROCK

DISTANCE: 9.5KM

DIFFICULTY: MODERATE

TIME: 4 HOURS

This circular route in the western Mournes gives a sampler of the incredible views in the region. The route ascends Hen, Cock and Pigeon Rock Mountains, using open mountain terrain, before going down through a valley to the starting car park. Expect stunning views and a great sense of accomplishment at the end of the walk.

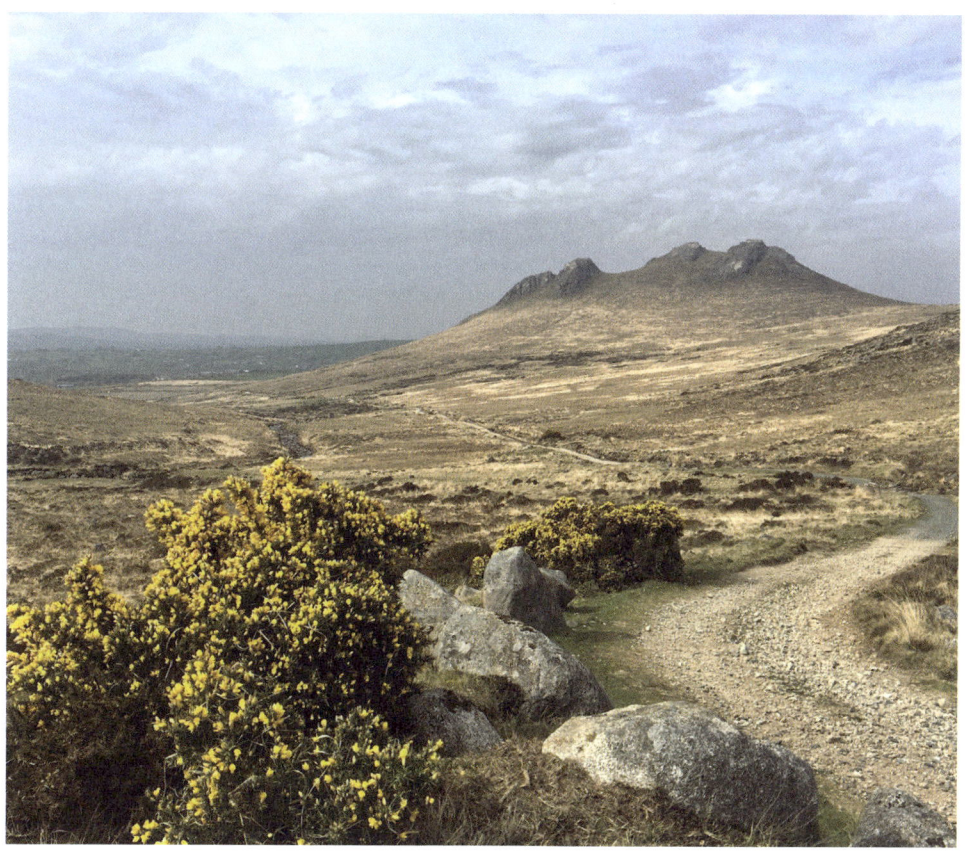

CAUSEWAY COAST WAY, CO. ANTRIM

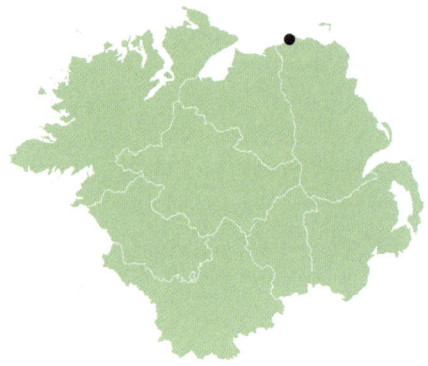

DISTANCE: 16KM

DIFFICULTY: EASY

TIME: 4–5 HOURS

The Causeway Coast Way follows Northern Ireland's most celebrated and dramatic stretch of coastline, which runs between Ballycastle and Portstewart. It is a beautiful part of the country and one that you really need to put on your bucket list if you haven't been already. The path extends for 51km (32 miles) over easy walking terrain of clifftops, beaches, promenades and occasional country roads.

The walk can be done in either direction and most people do it in sections over several days.

Some of the highlights include:

+ The Giant's Causeway
+ The medieval ruins of Dunluce Castle
+ The rope bridge connecting the mainland with the tiny island of Carrick-a-Rede
+ Bushmills Distillery
+ Rathlin Island, which can be visited from Ballycastle

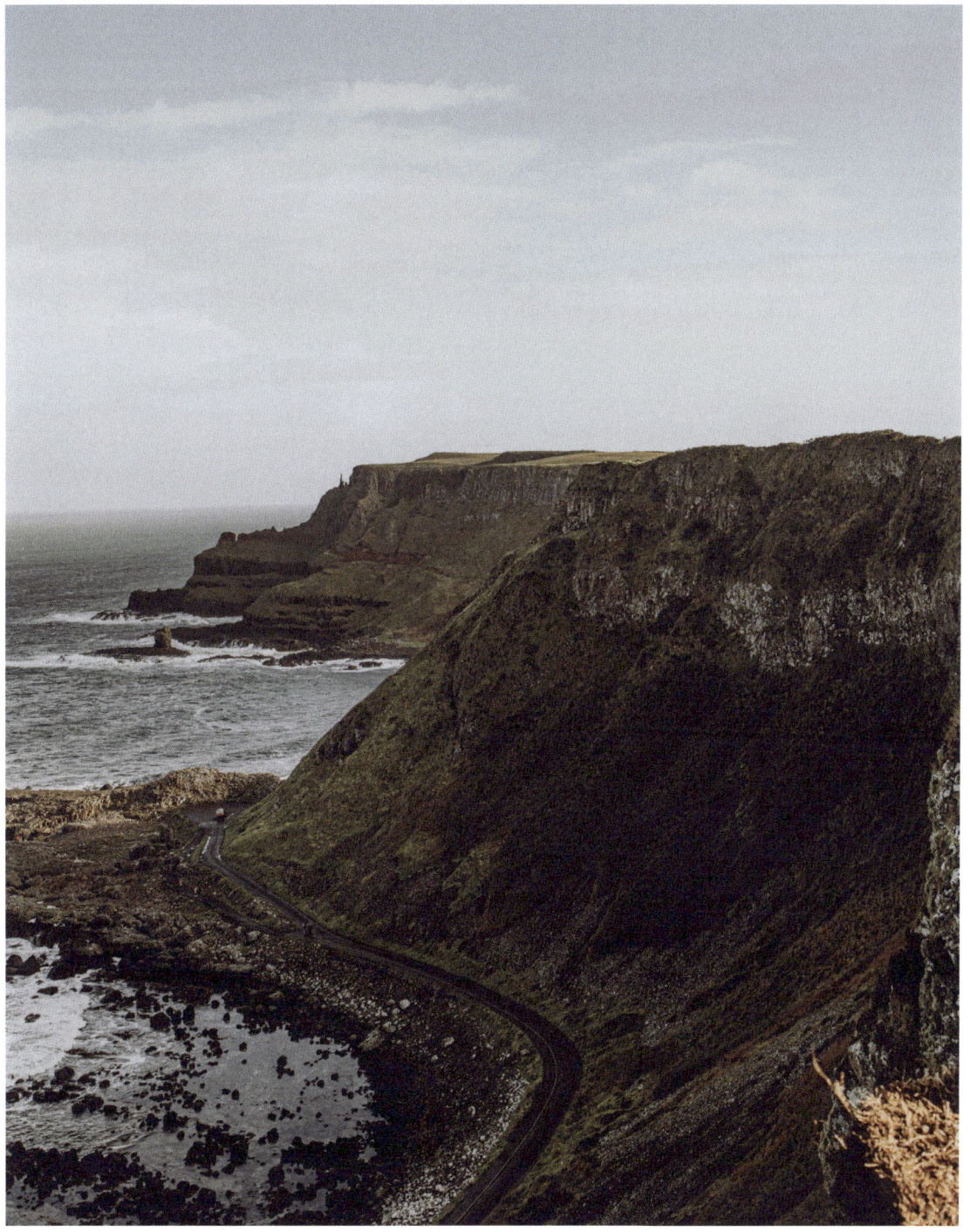

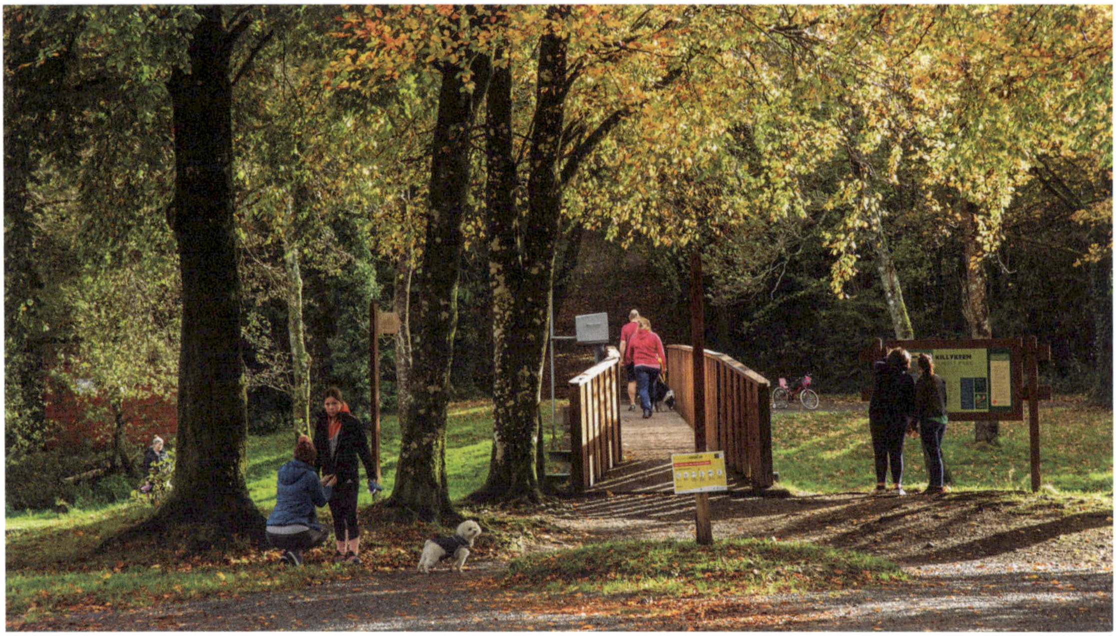

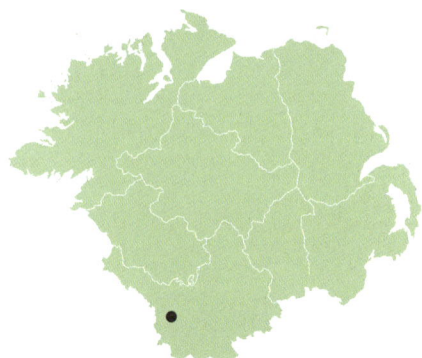

KILLYKEEN NATIONAL PARK, CO. CAVAN

DISTANCE: 3KM

DIFFICULTY: EASY

TIME: 1 HOUR

This is another great family walk. Killykeen Forest Park is a beautiful forest park wrapped around the idyllic Lough Oughter lake system and there are several woodland walking routes you can choose from.

This one, which will take you on a 1-hour lakeland scenery experience walk, is a 3km forest loop by tranquil Lough Oughter. Following lush forest paths, you'll spot tree species like Norway spruce, Sitka Spruce, ash, oak and beech and, of course, stunning lakeshore views.

This is not only a great area for walking; you can bring bikes and if the weather is good it is a great place to swim too!

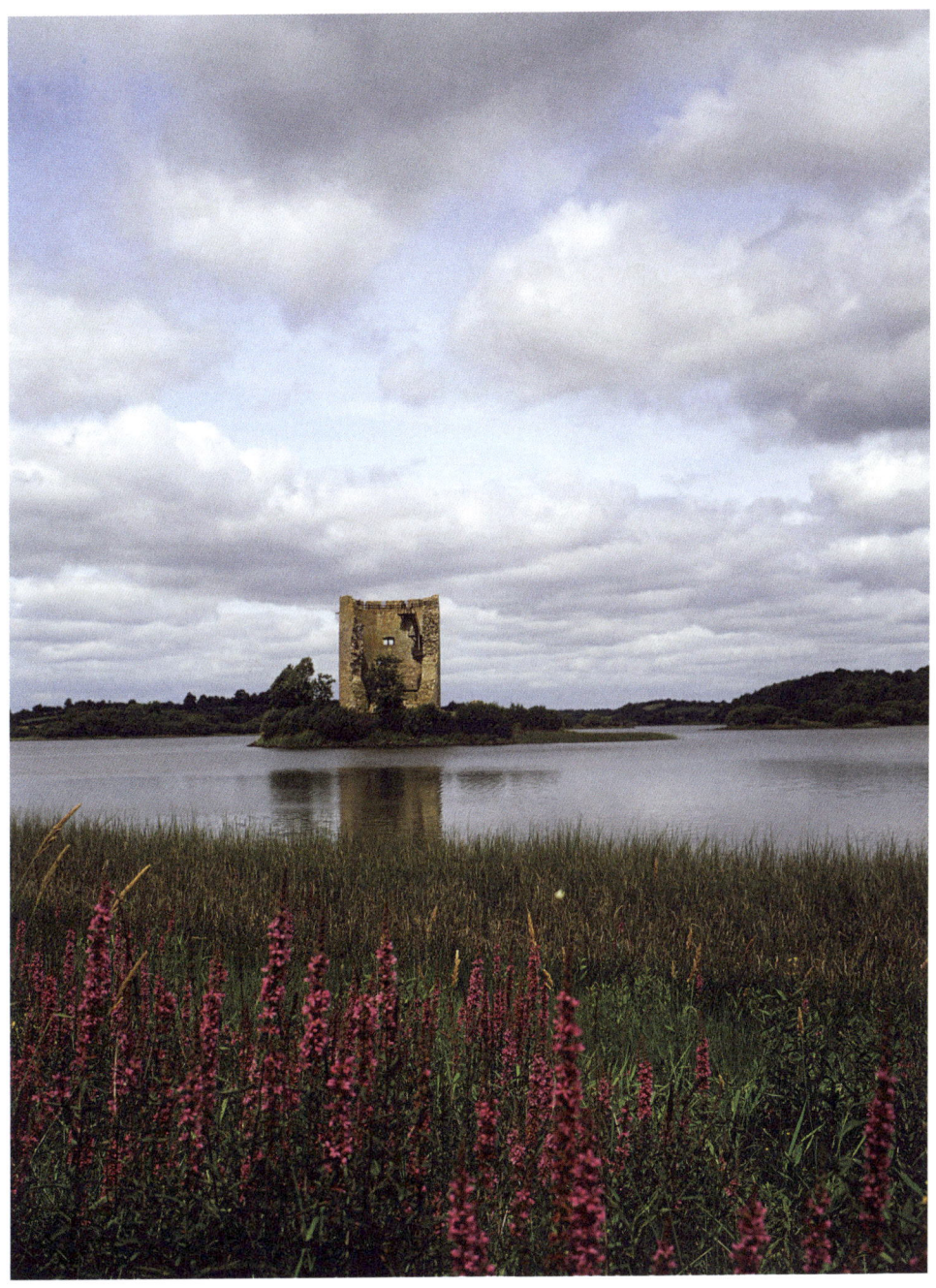

SLIEVE LEAGUE CLIFFS, CO. DONEGAL

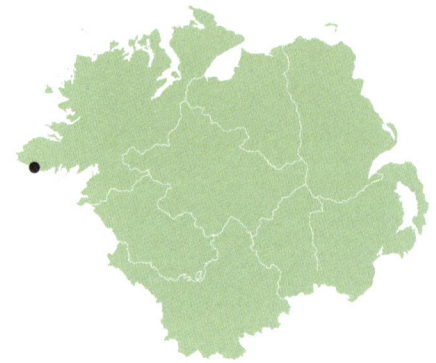

DISTANCE: 3KM

DIFFICULTY: EASY

TIME: 2–3 HOURS/4–5 HOURS

One of the most Instagrammable hikes in Ireland, this is a stunning walk that delivers incredible views. Ideally, take the Pilgrim's Path to the clifftops (see below). To get there, start by following a narrow road up from Teelin village for about a kilometre to where the road ends in a car park and trailhead. As always, make sure you don't leave any valuables in your car. The Pilgrim's Path is around 3km in length and it's around 2–3 hours out and back along a rough path worn into the mountain.

Another option is to continue up One Man's Pass, along the cliffs and down to Bunglas and either walk back along the country roads or try to arrange a taxi. This full-length walk will take around 4–5 hours.

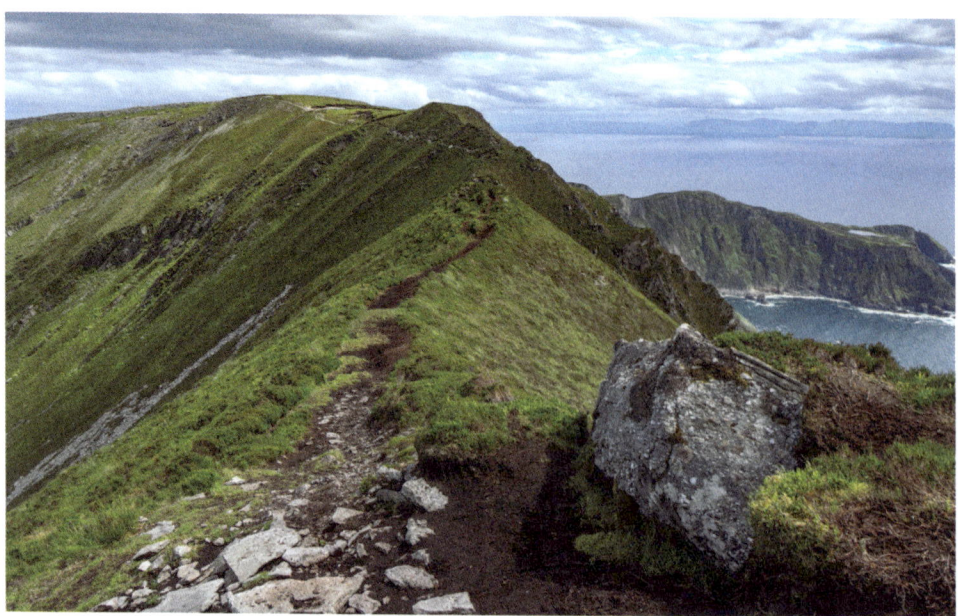

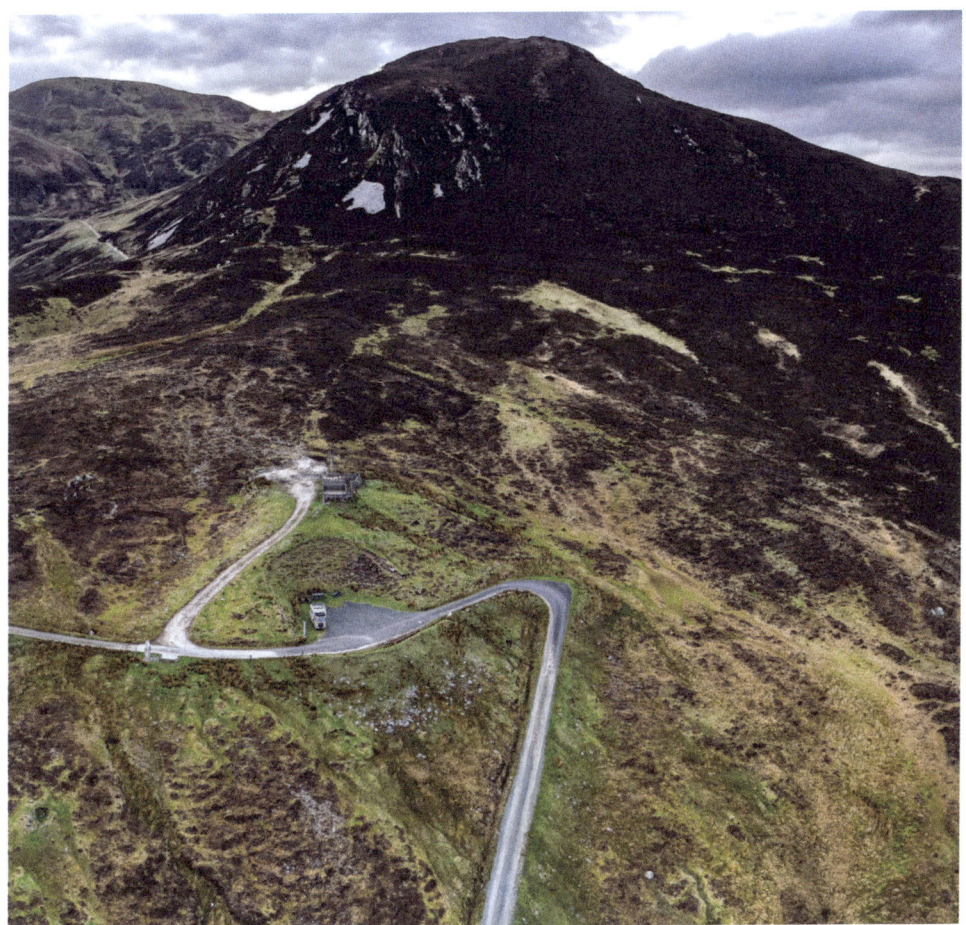

SLIEVE LEAGUE PILGRIMS' PATH

> DISTANCE: 2.8KM
>
> DIFFICULTY: MODERATE
>
> DURATION: 1.5 HOURS

The Slieve League Cliffs are among the highest sea cliffs in Europe, and if you're looking for a walk that will take your breath away, this is it. Starting out steady, the path soon becomes rocky as it winds its way up to about 420 metres. Along the way, you'll be treated to incredible Atlantic views; racing skies, which can change from pale blue to deep grey in minutes; and craggy, rocky landscapes that tumble down to the water. The weather can change quickly so make sure you come well prepared with the right clothing and suitable footwear.

'STAIRWAY TO HEAVEN', CO. FERMANAGH

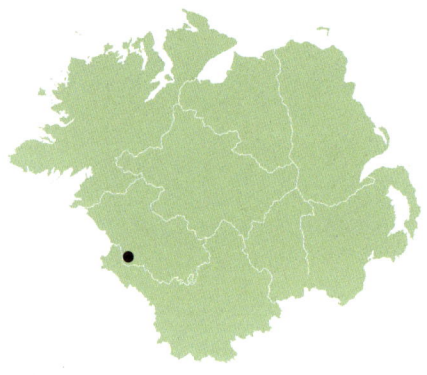

DISTANCE: 11 KM

DIFFICULTY: MODERATE

TIME: 3 HOURS

Situated on the doorstep of the Marble Arch Caves, the Cuilcagh Boardwalk Trail (also known as the 'Stairway to Heaven') has become famous over the last few years. It's about 16km from Enniskillen, or a 2-hour drive from Belfast, or a 1 hour 40-minute drive from Derry.

The boardwalk trail is a round trip of 11km from the car park to the viewing platform, at the top of the mountain. It's challenging in places, but take a break when you need to.

The walk begins along a gravel path from the car park which is around 4km in length. It is a great warm-up before you begin to climb the stairs of the boardwalk. This section of the trail is constructed out of wooden planks, forming a boardwalk that protects the delicate blanket bog underneath. Once you reach the boardwalk, you will then begin the ascent of Cuilcagh Mountain, which is 1.5km long.

As you approach the peak, a steep set of steps leads to the famous viewing platform, which provides breathtaking views of the nearby lowlands and a chance for a well-earned rest before beginning your descent.

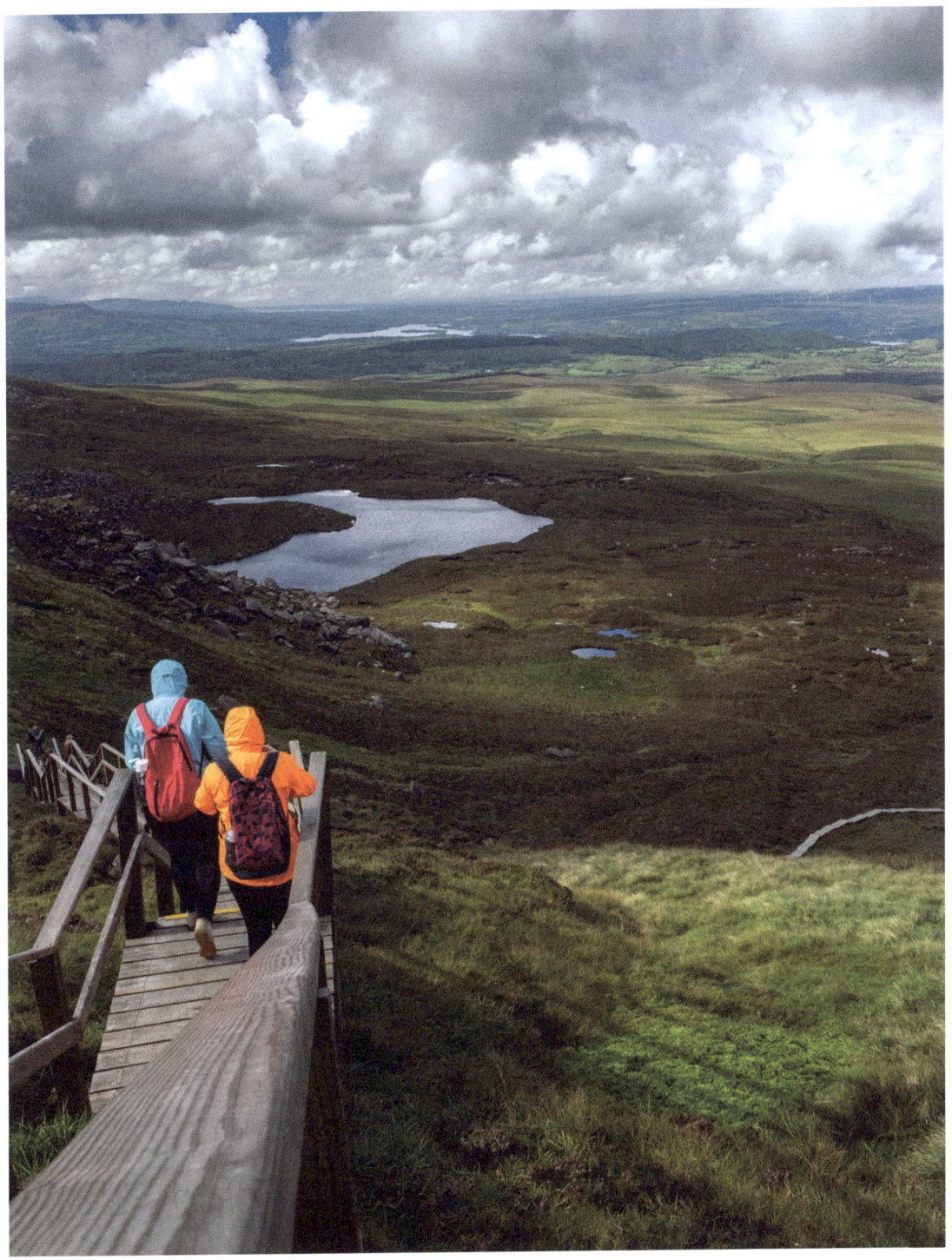

GOBBINS CLIFF PATH, CO. ANTRIM

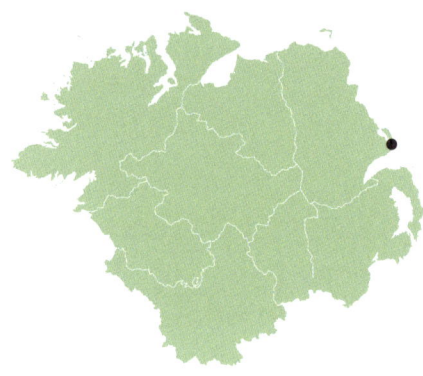

DISTANCE: 5KM

DIFFICULTY: HARD

DURATION: AROUND 2.5 HOURS, GUIDED WALKING

Wrapped around the sea cliffs of County Antrim, the Gobbins is the only guided adventure walk of its kind in Europe. This incredible path snakes through dramatic tubular bridges and smugglers' caves, and above crashing waves, and is a truly elemental experience. First opened in 1902 and designed by enterprising Edwardian engineer Berkeley Deane Wise, the Gobbins was reopened in 2015 and it remains as captivating as ever. From your first step through Wise's Eye at the path's mouth, you can't help but marvel at the incredible engineering that brought this path to life over a century ago.

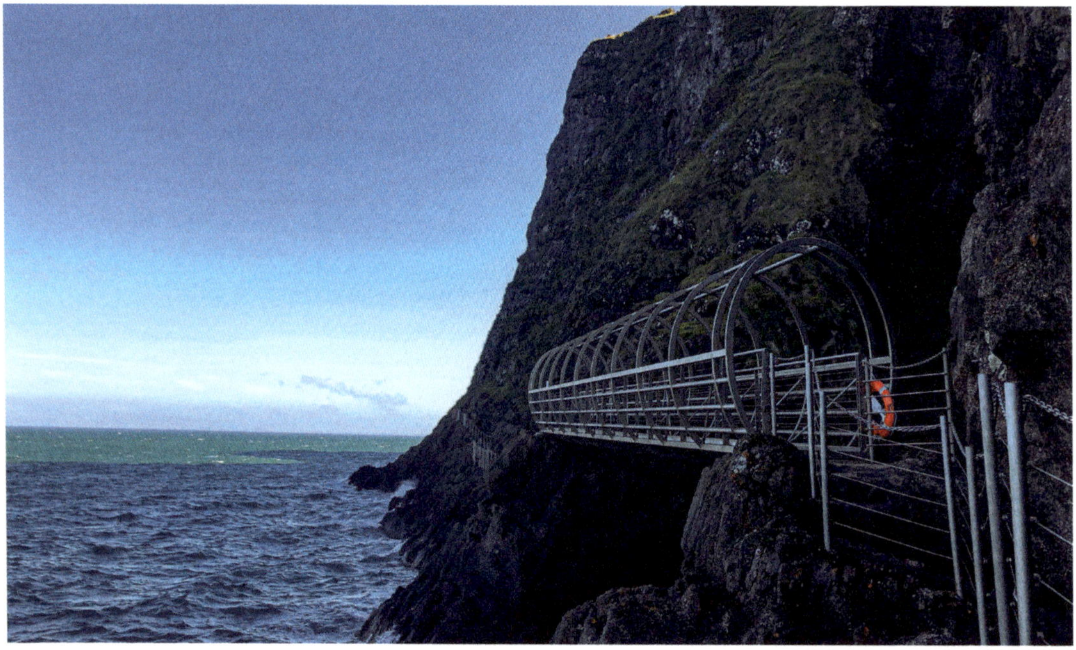

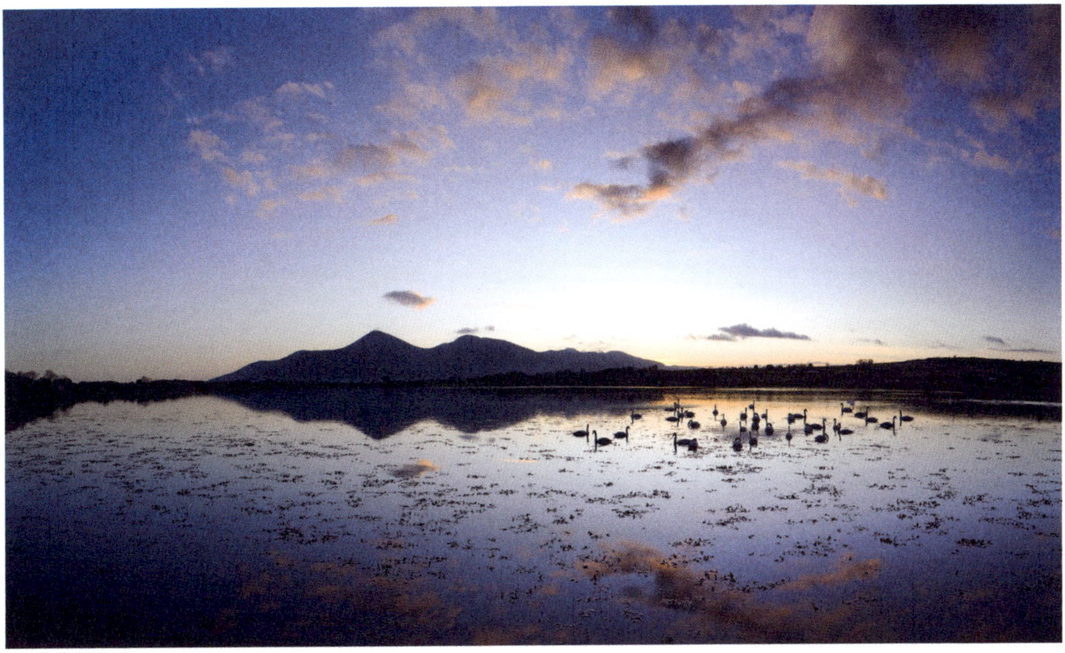

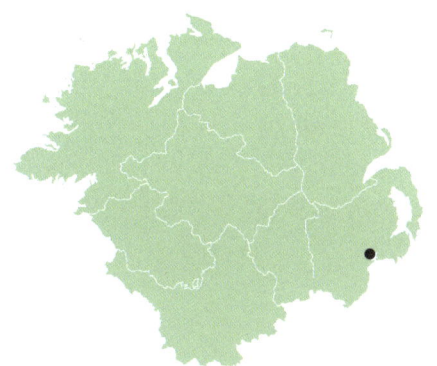

DUNDRUM BAY AND
THE MOURNE MOUNTAINS, COUNTY DOWN

DISTANCE: 2.5KM

DIFFICULTY: EASY

DURATION: 1.5 HOURS

Part of the longer Lecale Way walk, the Dundrum Coastal Path is a short and pleasant walk with lovely panoramas across Dundrum Inner Bay to the grey-blue beauty of the Mourne Mountains. The area is popular with birdwatchers. The path weaves along an old railway line through grassland, by pools and sand dunes, and offers beautiful views of the ruins of medieval Dundrum Castle. This walk is stunning at high tide, but birdwatchers should wait until the tide is out, when the best of the birdlife can be spotted along the estuarine sands.

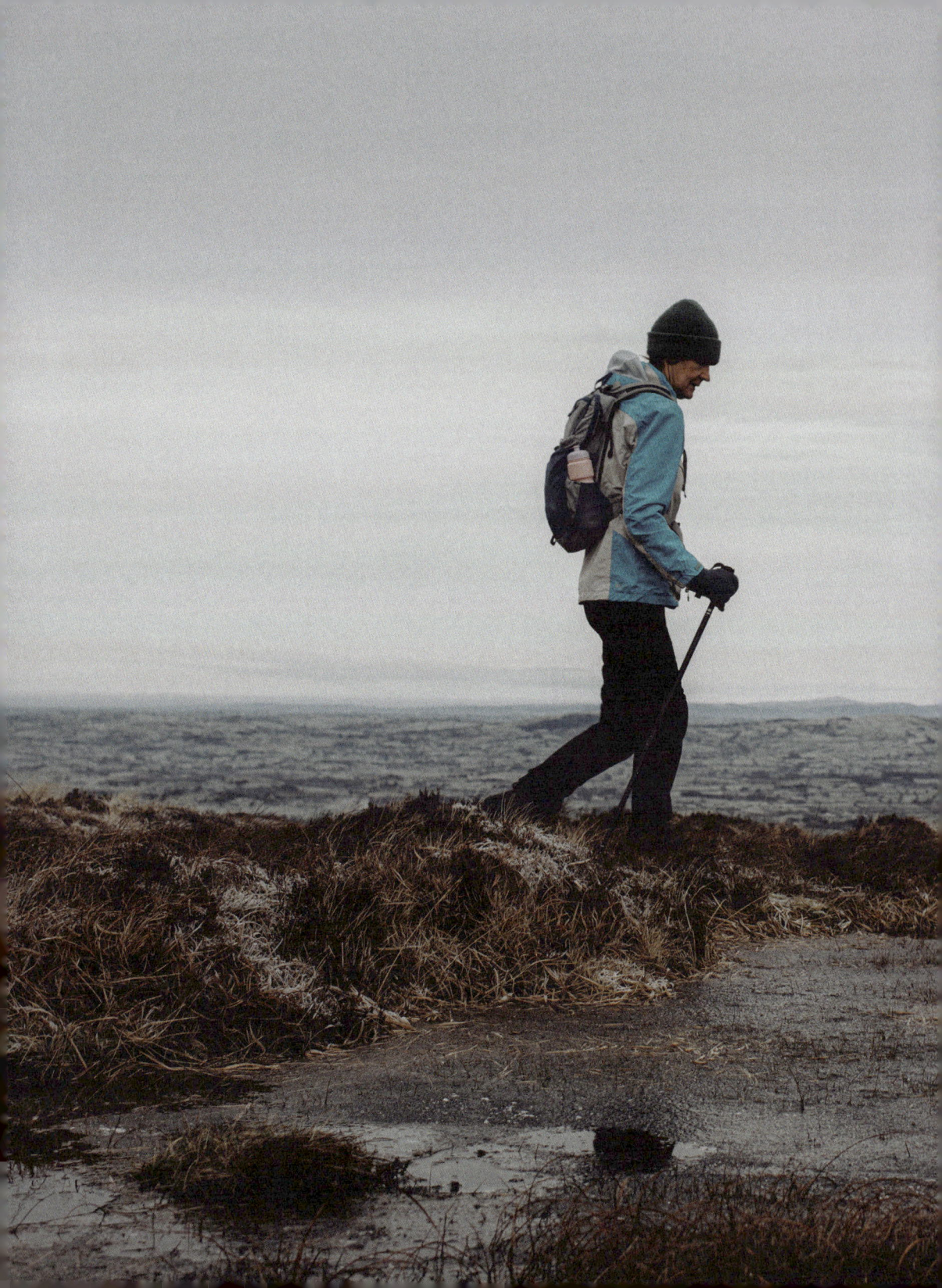

FAMILY WALKS

I love to see families out walking and exploring together. It's never too early to introduce your children to the joys of walking and it is so important to create those healthy habits at a young age. I've listed here some of my favourite family walks – but there are so many others across Ireland. Even if your kids or teenagers complain about going, they'll almost always enjoy the walk once you're underway and will have a sense of accomplishment at the end. Older children and teenagers might like to help plan the route and enjoy the challenge of trying to complete it in a particular time frame. All ages can try to identify some of the nature along the way too. Best of all, these are great free activities for all to enjoy all year round!

+ Crone Wood, Wicklow
+ Howth Cliff Walk
+ Torc Waterfall, Killarney
+ Kilclooney Wood, Waterford
+ Ticknock and Fairy Castle, Dublin
+ Ballinastoe Woods, Wicklow
+ Glendalough Spinc Trail, Wicklow
+ Devil's Glen, Wicklow
+ Avondale Forest Park, Wicklow

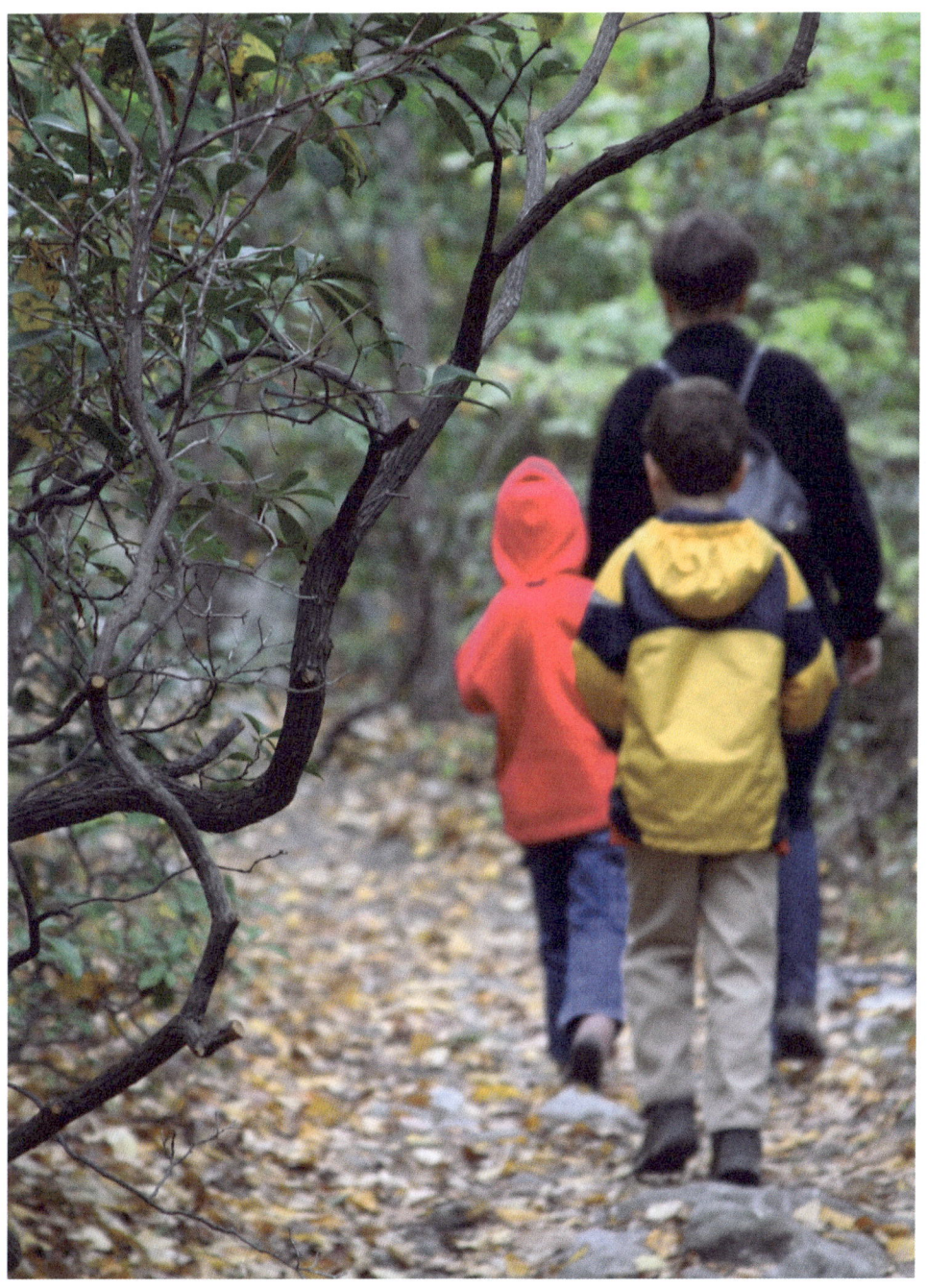

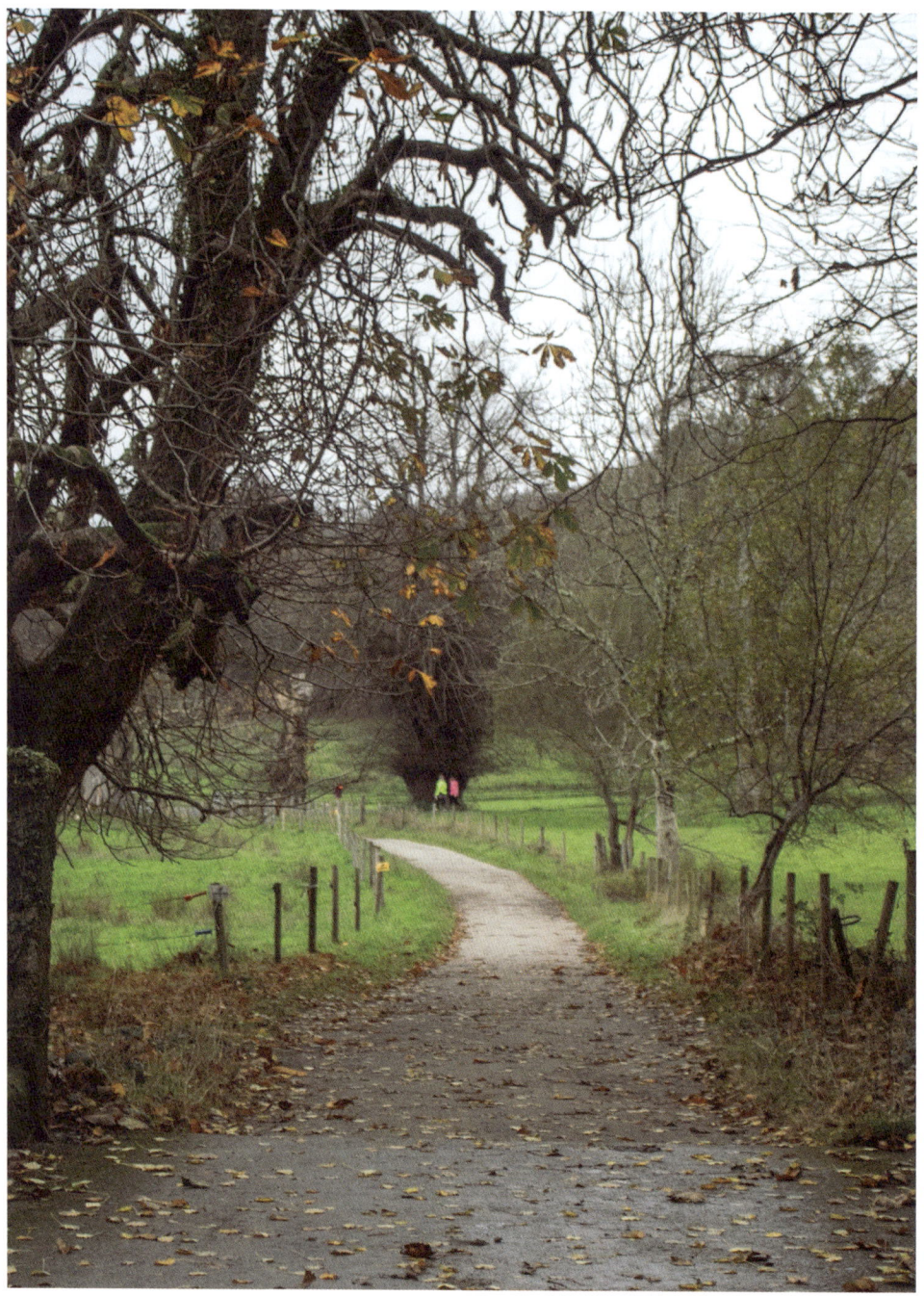

COUNTRY HOUSE WALKS

Ireland has such a rich history of historic houses, castles and estates, and I love exploring them and their grounds. There is often a choice of walks at country houses, all clearly signposted, and there can also be the bonus of visiting the house itself – and sometimes a cafe afterwards too! I hope you'll enjoying checking some of these off your list.

+ Carton House, Kildare
+ Newbridge House, Donabate
+ Castlefreke, Cork
+ Muckross House, Killarney
+ Phoenix Park, Dublin
+ Mount Congreve, Waterford

BEACH WALKS

Give me a windy, wintry day, a good jacket and a
good walk, and I am a happy man! Walking by the
sea is both hugely enjoyable, and brilliant for your
body and mind (see pages 134–6). We have some
of the most beautiful beaches in the world, often
very close by – I would encourage you to get out
and enjoy them year-round. The list below is just
a small sample of some of the beach walks I love
the best.

+ Inch Strand, Kerry
+ Donabate, Dublin
+ Inchydoney, Cork
+ Brittas Bay, Wicklow
+ Long Strand, Cork

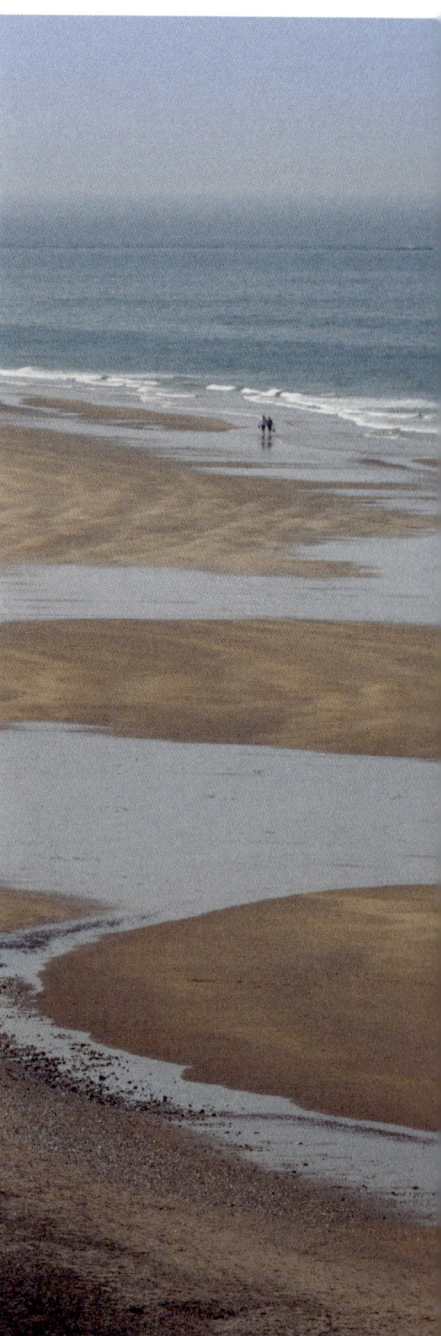

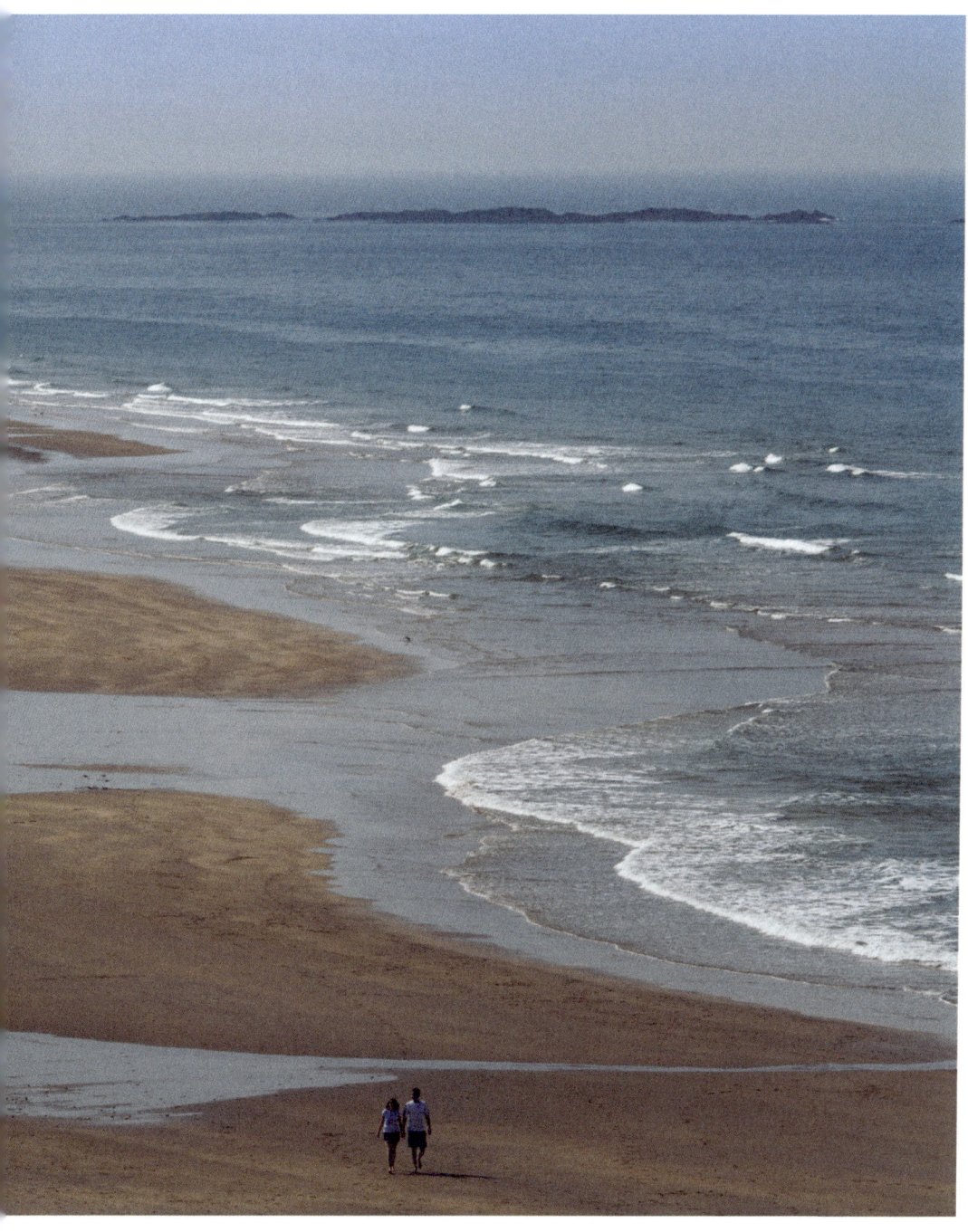

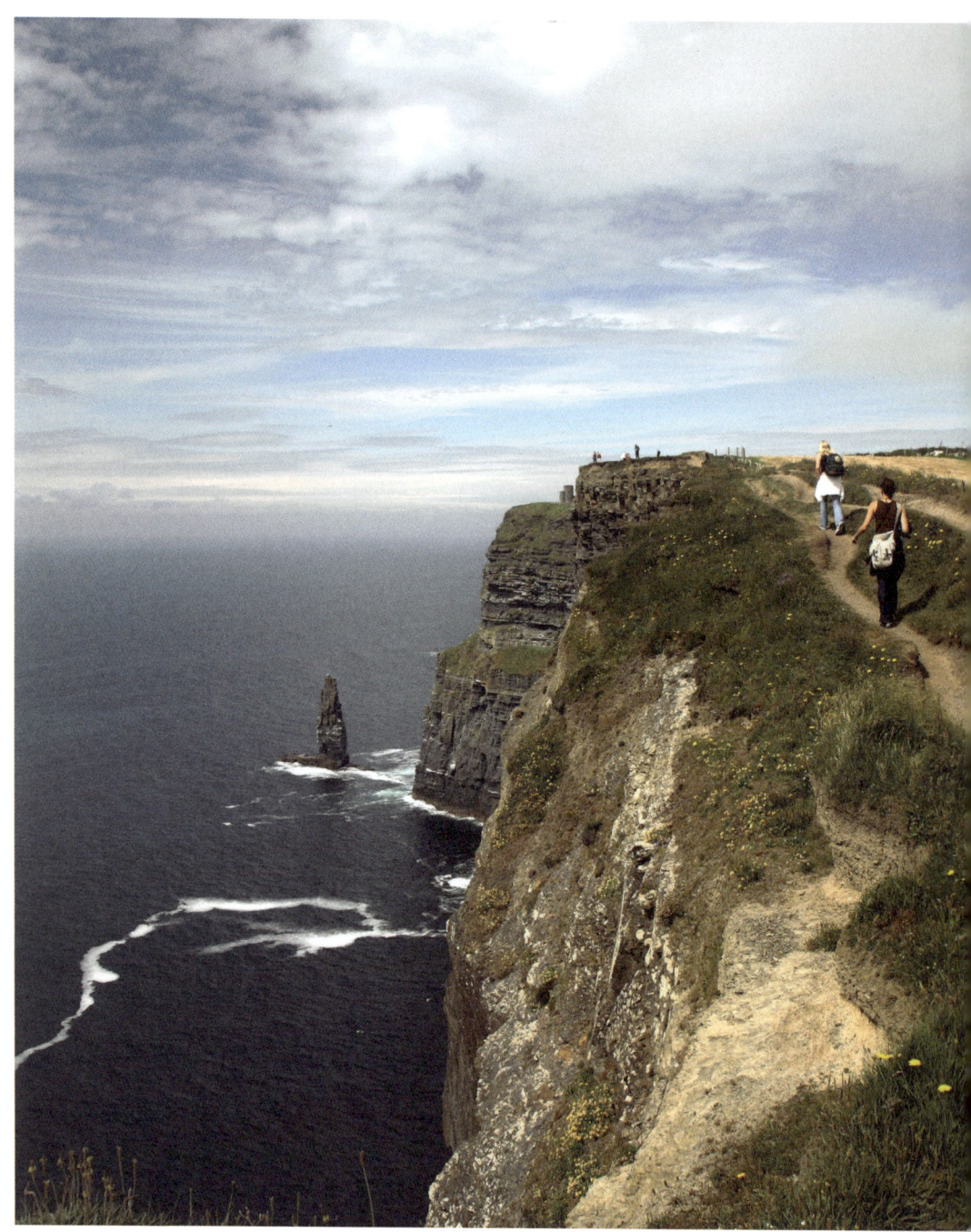

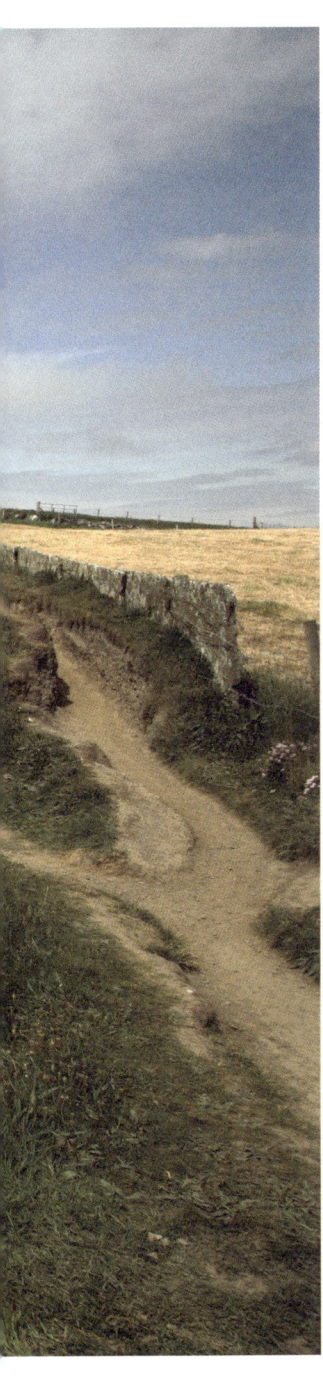

CLIFF WALKS

Cliff walks offer incredible views and all the benefits of sea air, sometimes with a challenging walk too. They often follow historic routes that have been there for hundreds of years, and there are few better places for spotting some amazing sea life.

+ Glencolmcille Loop, Donegal
+ Howth Cliff Walk, Dublin
+ Bray to Greystones, Wicklow (currently closed, but due to reopen soon)
+ Ardmore Cliff Walk, Waterford
+ Cliffs of Moher Coastal Walk, Clare
+ Sheep's Head, Cork
+ Ballycotton Cliff Walk, Cork
+ Bray Head Loop, Kerry
+ Ballybunion Cliff Path, Kerry
+ Portrane Cliff Walk, Dublin

BIBLIOGRAPHY

Asthma+Lung UK. 'Physical activity and your lungs'. *Asthma+LungUK* [online]. https://www. asthmaandlung.org.uk/living-with/keeping-active/physical-activity

Carreño, A., Fontdecaba, E., Izquierdo-Font, A., Enciso, O., Daunis-i-Estadella, P., Mateu-Figueras, G., Palarea-Albaladejo, J., Mireia, G., Vendrell, C., Lloveras, M., San, J., Gómez Mestres, S., Minuto, S., Lloret, J. (2023). 'Blue prescription: A pilot study of health benefits for oncological patients of a short program of activities involving the sea.' *Heliyon.* 9. e17713. doi: 10.1016/j.heliyon.2023.e17713

Cox, D., Shanahan, D., Hudson, H., Plummer, K., Siriwardena, G., Fuller, R., Anderson, K., Hancock, S., Gaston, K. (2017). 'Doses of Neighborhood Nature: The Benefits for Mental Health of Living with Nature.' *BioScience.* doi: 10.1093/biosci/biw173.

del Pozo Cruz, B., Ahmadi, M., Naismith, S.L., Stamatakis, E. (2022). 'Association of Daily Step Count and Intensity With Incident Dementia in 78,430 Adults Living in the UK.' *JAMA Neurol.*, 79(10):1059–1063. doi: 10.1001/jamaneurol.2022.2672

Erickson, K.I., Voss, M.W., Prakash, R.S., Basak, C., Szabo, A., Chaddock, L., Kim, J.S., Heo, S., Alves, H., White, S.M., Wojcicki, T.R., Mailey, E., Vieira, V.J., Martin, S.A., Pence, B.D., Woods, J.A., McAuley, E., Kramer, A.F. (2011). 'Exercise training increases size of hippocampus and improves memory.' *Proceedings of the National Academy of Sciences of the United States of America.* 108(7):3017–22. doi: 10.1073/pnas.1015950108

Harvard School of Public Health. (2021). 'The health benefits of trees.' *Harvard School of Public Health* [online]. https://hsph.harvard.edu/news/the-health-benefits-of-trees/

Hunter, M.C.R., Gillespie, B. W., Chen, S. Y.-P. (2019). 'Urban Nature Experiences Reduce Stress in the Context of Daily Life Based on Salivary Biomarkers'. *Frontiers in Psychology.* 10. doi: 10.3389/fpsyg.2019.00722

Kalyani, R.R., Corriere, M., Ferrucci, L. (2014). 'Age-related and disease-related muscle loss: the effect of diabetes, obesity, and other diseases.' *The Lancet. Diabetes & endocrinology*, 2(10), 819–829. doi: 10.1016/S2213-8587(14)70034-8

Krall, E.A., Dawson-Hughes, B. (1994). 'Walking is related to bone density and rates of bone loss.' *American Journal of Medicine*, 96(1):20–6. doi: 10.1016/0002-9343(94)90111-2

LeWine, H.E. (2024). 'The importance of stretching.' *Harvard Health Publishing, Harvard Medical School* [online]. https://www.health.harvard.edu/staying-healthy/the-importance-of-stretching

Murtagh, E.M., Nichols, L., Mohammed, M.A., Holder, R., Nevill, A.M., Murphy, M.H. (2015). 'The effect of walking on risk factors for cardiovascular disease: An updated systematic review and meta-analysis of randomised control trials.' *Preventive Medicine*, 72, 34–43. doi: 10.1016/j.ypmed.2014.12.041

Oh, H., & Taylor, A. H. (2013). 'A brisk walk, compared with being sedentary, reduces attentional bias and chocolate cravings among regular chocolate eaters with different body mass.' *Appetite*, 71, 144–149. doi: 10.1016/j.appet.2013.07.01

Ratey, J. J. (2019). 'Can exercise help treat anxiety?' *Harvard Health Publishing, Harvard Medical School* [online]. https://www.health.harvard.edu/blog/can-exercise-help-treat-anxiety-2019102418096

Strain, T., Flaxman, S., Guthold, R., Semenova, E., Cowan, M., Riley, L.M., Bull, F., Stevens, G.A., & Garcia, L. (2024). 'National, regional, and global trends in insufficient physical activity among adults from 2000 to 2022: a pooled analysis of 507 population-based surveys with 5·7 million participants.' *The Lancet. Global Health*, 12(8), e1232-e1243. doi: 10.1016/S2214-109X(24)00150-5

Ungvari, Z., Fazekas-Pongor, V., Csiszar, A., & Kunutsor, S.K. (2023). 'The multifaceted benefits of walking for healthy aging: from Blue Zones to molecular mechanisms.' *GeroScience*, 45(6), 3211–3239. doi: 10.1007/s11357-023-00873-8

University Hospitals (2024). 'Breathe Your Way to Better Health & Less Stress.' *University Hospitals* [online]. https://www.uhhospitals.org/blog/articles/2024/02/breathe-your-way-to-better-health-and-less-stress

ACKNOWLEDGEMENTS

Two words really, thank you.

Thank you to everyone who believes in the work that I do

To the team at NK Management

To the team at Gill

To my friends

To my family

And to you, the reader: thank you for wanting to be healthier, and for believing in me and in what I do so that we can do it together.

IMAGE CREDITS

NOTES

NOTES

NOTES

NOTES

NOTES

NOTES